Age Right

TURN BACK THE CLOCK WITH A PROVEN, PERSONALIZED ANTIAGING PROGRAM

Karlis Ullis, M.D.

with Greg Ptacek

SIMON & SCHUSTER

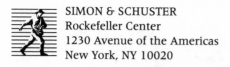 SIMON & SCHUSTER
Rockefeller Center
1230 Avenue of the Americas
New York, NY 10020

SIMON & SCHUSTER and colophon are registered trademarks of
Simon & Schuster Inc.

Designed by Meryl Sussman Levavi/digitext, inc.

Manufactured in the United States of America

10   9   8   7   6   5   4   3   2   1

Library of Congress Cataloging-in-Publication Data
Ullis, Karlis.
     Age right : turn back the clock with a proven, personalized
  antiaging program / Karlis Ullis, with Greg Ptacek.
        p.   cm.
     Includes bibliographical references and index.
     1. Rejuvenation—Popular works.   2. Aging—Prevention—
  Popular works.   I. Ptacek, Greg.   II. Title.
  RA776.75.U54   1999
  613—dc21   98-44889   CIP
  ISBN 0-684-84197-5

Acknowledgments

My first thank-yous go to the individuals who helped conceive and provide the impetus to write this book: coauthor Greg Ptacek for the idea, Yvette Harper for the inspiration to follow through, and Ethlie Ann Vare for her invaluable assistance in the initial stages of the book. Thanks also to my two key UCLA research assistants, Kishan Patel and Kira Molas, for dredging the depths of the UCLA biomedical library for research documents; my office staff personnel, June Sutikno and Kate Eisenhauer, for holding down the fort while I put in due diligence for this book; my brother, John J. Ullis, who at all times was available to provide the best and latest computer systems and support; Sydny Miner for insightful editing; Rose Ann Ferrick for her precise and thoughtful copyediting and Harvey Klinger for embracing the project and finding a home for its publication.

Special thanks also go to:

◆ the athletes and coaches I have had the pleasure of working with over these last two decades at UCLA, the Santa Monica Track Club, and the international Olympic teams: Steve Lewis, Danny Everett, Michael Marsh, Gail Devers, Valerie Brisco, Mike Tully, Mike Powell, Willie Banks, Kevin Young, Reggie Miller, John Brenner, Flo-Jo Joyner, Al Joyner, Jackie

Joyner-Kersee, Jon Smith, Art Venegas, and Joe Douglas. Their dedication to pushing the boundaries of human athletic endurance laid the foundation for the theories of antiaging presented in this book. Thanks also to the Olympic teams of Latvia, El Salvador, and Sierra Leone for incredibly exciting experiences at the games in Seoul, Albertville, Barcelona, and Lillehammer, and to Latvian bobsled team members, their coach Zintis Ekmanis, and triple jumper Maris Bruziks for their insight into the world of the Soviet sports machine;

◆ my sports medicine and sports science colleagues at UCLA for their scientific knowledge and Jo Ann Dawson, M.D., for her understanding and support of my time demands;

◆ the members of the Los Angeles Gerontology Research Group, especially L. Stephen Coles, M.D., Ph.D., for his amazing capacity to gather the latest information about the significant and rapidly moving science of antiaging clinical medicine, genetics, and biotechnology; Ray Sahelian, M.D., for his understanding of the world of DHEA, pregnenolone, and melatonin; Jeffrey Bland, Ph.D., for his inspirational seminars on functional medicine and nutritional biochemistry;

◆ my daughters, Sarina and Dzintra, whose vitality led me to the extropy concepts about cellular organization, growth, development, and aging;

◆ the practitioners in the healing arts who gave me new and different ways to understand the biomechanics of the human body involving Rolfing, Heller, Alexander, Feldenkreis, acupuncture, Neuro-Muscular Therapy (NMT), manual-physical therapy, and the other physical medicine rehabilitation disciplines;

◆ the Growth Hormone Research Society, including Peter Sonksen, M.D., and the other members, especially Bengt-Ake Bengtsson, M.D., of Sweden who allowed me to roam around in the most amazing human growth hormone laboratory in the world;

◆ and Amy Wong for technical support, B. A. Kus for moral support, Kimberly Ball for her precise transcriptions, Maile Speetjens for unending moral support and Cristiana Paul, M.S., for her nutritional insights.

To my two beautiful and wonderful
daughters, Sarina and Dzintra, incredible
examples of boundless extropic energy

Contents

Part III: Customizing Your Antiaging Regimen

Part IV: Antiaging Resources

APPENDICES

Introduction

I am making several assumptions about you.

Assumption #1: You are among those of us who think that growing old is anything but graceful. Despite the best efforts of Hollywood and Madison Avenue to market middle age as the prime of your life, in reality there's nothing sexy about wrinkles, graying hair, spreading middles, sagging jowls, fading vision, diminishing sex drive, and loss of memory.

Assumption #2: You have already spent more money than you would like to admit on health clubs, diet plans, and maybe even cosmetic surgery to look younger. You are not alone. Last year Americans spent more than $35 billion on trying to lose weight and underwent more than 400,000 cosmetic surgical procedures.

Assumption #3: You would be willing to spend time and effort if you could actually *feel* younger. Now there's the challenge. Is there any way to actually stop—and reverse—nature's aging clock? Ten years ago the answer was a resounding *no*. Today, thanks to remarkably practical advances in antiaging medicine, the answer is yes, decidedly *yes*.

This book provides a step-by-step approach to creating an antiaging program that can actually slow and even reverse the physical and mental deterioration associated with aging. Let me put that another way: With the advanced antiaging system presented here, it is possible to not only *stay* young but to *grow younger*.

You may have heard that claim before. But this book is different from any other because it approaches antiaging from a new perspective: Not everyone ages in the same way. Our unique genetic blueprints and lifetime experiences mean that the process of aging affects each of us in different ways. Therefore, we cannot be treated in the same way. This concept is vitally important in creating an effective antiaging strategy, but it has been ignored so far. Why? For one thing, it is easier to tell everybody the same thing: Take a handful of superhormone X and call me in the morning.

Age Right is the first book to actually show you how to develop an antiaging regimen that fits your individual aging profile. Your program will be designed for your aging characteristics, utilizing the same approach I use with patients who visit my antiaging clinic and taking into consideration your biochemical profile and factors that include age, medical history, body type, gender, and lifestyle.

By the end of this book you will have an actual antiaging day planner with a regimen of supplements that include phytonutrients, vitamins, antioxidants, "smart drugs," those substances that enhance mental performance, herbs, and amino acids. Combined with a training or exercise program and diet and lifestyle recommendations, this customized regimen will provide you with the tools to counter age-related disabilities from creaky joints to decreasing mental performance. You will improve your ability to relax and sleep, enhance your immune function, lose excess weight and keep it off, heighten sexual ability and performance, increase bone density and lung capacity, and enhance skin and muscle tone. By any measurement you will look and feel younger.

As an attending physician at five Olympic Games, I developed a results-oriented therapy that bridges the gap between scientifically solid advanced research and everyday application. Your antiaging program will incorporate the same cutting-edge techniques that the world's best athletes use to increase their performance.

My strategies for antiaging were developed during my twenty-year tenure at UCLA's Sports Medicine and Rehabilitation Clinics where I treated many of these gifted athletes on the playing field and in the gym. We spent hours together discussing their training secrets. And that's when I began to observe that the symptoms these elite athletes were experiencing from overtraining were physiologically identical to those of my middle-age patients in my private practice.

Could the same treatments that helped the world's best athletes recover their health be applied to my patients experiencing the first effects of advanced aging? The answer was a startling *yes*.

In *Age Right* you will learn that as children and young adults we had a natural repair process called *anabolic drive* which continuously regenerated body tissue. Gradually, we lose this rejuvenating capacity and develop numerous conditions associated with aging: obesity, heart disease, and Alzheimer's, to name a few. But thanks to recent advances in antiaging medicine, we can actually regain that anabolic drive by replenishing depleted levels of hormones, the fluids that regulate our organs and tissues, and neurotransmitters, the brain's chemical messengers.

We are the first generation in history to have a say in our biological destiny. Advances in biotechnology and genetics research are ushering in a new age of antiaging therapy. To take full advantage of the wonders that await us in the next century, we must bridge the gap with the treatments available now that can dramatically enhance the quality of our lives. *Age Right* provides the answers to holding back the hands of time.

How to Use This Book

This book is designed to create an antiaging regimen specific to your aging pathway. Using a series of questionnaires and tests, we will pinpoint exactly where your weakest areas of defense are and supply you with the weapons to combat the effects of aging.

Parts One and Four provide valuable background information. Part One explains how and why we age and current theories of aging. Part Four provides a detailed guide that makes sense of all the antiaging products on the market today, a guide to antiaging foods, and a look at antiaging treatments on the horizon. But if you're in a hurry to get started on your antiaging regimen, skip these chapters for now.

The core of *Age Right* are Parts Two and Three. This is where you will discover your aging pathway and your current biological age. With this data you can be shown how to build an antiaging regimen with strategies that address your individual strengths and weaknesses. You will also find appendices on supplements, diet, and exercise. Use these references to complement your antiaging day regimen.

It is always recommended that you consult with your physician before embarking on an unusual or vastly different health and fitness regimen.

This book is part of an ongoing study of applying advanced antiaging research to the general public. We would like to hear your thoughts and comments on the programs presented here. Contact us at:

Sports Medicine & Anti-Aging Medical Group
1807 Wilshire Blvd., Suite 205
Santa Monica, CA 90403
Phone: (310) 829-1990
Fax: (310) 829-5134
E-mail: kulllis@ucla.edu
Website: http://www.agingprevent.com

~ Part I ~

The Process
of Aging

~ 1 ~

Why We Age

For the human race long life is a recent development. Two thousand years ago the average citizen of the Roman Empire could expect to live only thirty years. The next eighteen centuries saw a slight improvement in life expectancy, increasing on the average of two days every year, so that by 1870 the average U.S. citizen could expect to live forty years. Then something extraordinary occurred. After centuries of achingly slow progress, longevity began to increase exponentially. Babies born only thirty-five years later, in 1915, could expect to live to fifty. In other words, what took the pre–Industrial Age to achieve in eighteen hundred years—that is, increasing the life span by ten years—took modern man only thirty-five years. And this trend has moved steadily upward so that the average baby born in the United States in the year 2000 can expect to live eighty years. (See Figure 1.)

There is no mystery as to why we have doubled our life expectancy in 130 years. The introduction of preventive medicine at the turn of the century beat into submission one of man's enemies: infectious disease. Deaths from contagious illnesses such as typhoid fever, diphtheria, influenza, dysentery, scarlet fever, and tuberculosis were appallingly high earlier in this century. It was not uncommon, for example, for fifteen hundred people to die weekly from infectious diseases in New York City in the late 1800s and early

Figure 1

Date	Average Life Expectancy (Years)
Prehistoric times	25
Roman Empire (0 A.D.)	30
1870 (U.S.)	40
1915	50
1930	60
1955	70
1992	75.8
1997	76
2000 (Estimated)	80

1900s. A worldwide influenza epidemic that struck in 1918 killed 500,000 people in the United States alone. Public health pioneers such as Dr. Sara Josephine Baker institutionalized simple but effective methods for extending longevity. Working first in Hell's Kitchen, the slums of New York, in the early 1900s, Baker and her team of nurses slashed the death rates by 80 percent for newborns by introducing tenement dwellers to such basic hygiene techniques as pasteurized milk and proper ventilation. Her programs were widely adopted by governments around the world.

As effective as these public hygiene crusades were, they did absolutely nothing to increase the life span. The genetically determined maximum life span for our species has remained depressingly stagnant. However, while a citizen of sixteenth-century Italy might have expected to live thirty-five years or so, that doesn't mean everyone keeled over by their fortieth birthday. History is filled with examples of individuals who had long lives even by our standards. For example, Luigi Cornaro, a sixteenth-century citizen of Venice, lived to ninety-eight and wrote an influential book about his longevity, *Discourses on the Temperate Life,* attributing it to temperance and an abstemious diet. (More on the correlation between aging and a calorie-restricted, nutrient-dense diet later.) Since the beginning of reliable recorded history, the maximum human life span has hovered around one hundred years.

The mystery about human mortality, then, is not why we live so long but rather why we don't live *longer.* What is in our inherent design that shuts down our biological systems at a genetically predetermined age? Why can't we live to 150, 200, or 500 years of age? The answer lies in a term that originated with gerontology, the scientific study of old age. Gerontologists use the word *senescence* to describe what we know as the physical and mental decline that accompanies old age. Amazingly, most living creatures do not senesce, that is, get more frail with age. Many species of insects, fish, and most invertebrates show the same biological age whether they are a minute or a millennium old. It turns out that humans, mammals, and other vertebrates have only recently developed genes that cause them to get old. This was not a case of evolutionary bad luck. Ironically, these old age genes helped the species survive and prosper.

Early on, our species picked up on the fact that its environment was no bed of roses. Between hungry predators and volcanic eruptions, it was faced with a constantly changing milieu. And as species went, ours, being the most complex physiologically, was the most vulnerable. To survive, man had to evolve constantly to meet the challenges. The choice came down to immortality (or at least very long age) or species variance (to introduce genetic changes as quickly as possible). This was hardly idle speculation. It is estimated that 99 percent of the species that ever lived on earth are now extinct. If the environment were a vacuum where no changes occurred, *homo sapiens* could have afforded the luxury of nonsenescence. Given the circumstances, our species had no choice but to hitch our wagon to the other vertebrates' and opt for a limited life span.

If the "Sophie's choice" was made for a limited life span, then the next question was when to end it. (Remember, the evolutionary objective was to introduce genetic changes as quickly as possible.) The answer, of course, is, as quickly as possible. And this is where senescence fits in. By our late twenties most of our major physiological systems peak. Biologically, that's just enough time to prepare our offspring for their reproductive years. Our ancient ancestors would protect and provide for their children until they were ready to have children of their own, a life span of twenty-five years, give or take a couple of years. Having marshaled our physiological resources for our reproductive years to ensure the survival of the next generation, Nature was essentially done with us after the age of twenty-five. If old age meant pain and suffering, hey, we as a species made the choice; at least ours was among the lucky 1 percent that continued to survive. If anything, the hangers-on of our species who refused to die after reproducing were a bit of a genetic nuisance, competing with fertile breeders for limited resources.

Which brings us back to the twentieth century. Having used the genius of our superior species to maximize our life expectancy, we find ourselves up against the ultimate brick wall—a genetically predetermined life span. But before you shrug and throw this book away, consider that there is nothing inevitable about aging. It is a *process;* in theory, elements of that process can be halted or even reversed. Exactly how the aging process works is a mystery, but already we know a lot about the individual elements. We know enough already to begin reversing the ravages of growing old. Senescence, you're about to meet your match.

2

How We Age

What do we mean by "age"? Yes, we all know to age means to grow older in years. But to a biologist, a measurement of aging based on your birth date is not very useful. After all, we all know of people who look ten years younger (or older) than their actual chronological age would indicate.

Having a practice in Los Angeles, my patients include many actors and models who *look* younger than their chronological age, but their beauty is literally skin deep, the result of skilled cosmetic surgery. They come to my clinic because despite laser wrinkle removals, breast implants, tummy tucks, buttock lifts, collagen injections, and ultrasound liposuction (among the more common procedures), they are beginning to suffer some of the "four D's" of advanced aging—discomfort, disability, drugs, and doctors. Their bodies are beginning to suffer the four main physiological changes that occur with aging: (1) decreased muscle mass, (2) decreased bone mass, (3) decreased water content, and (4) increased fat levels. As we will see, these changes are accompanied by a slew of undesirable symptoms. And much to their chagrin, my Hollywood patients know that the best cosmetic surgery money can buy does nothing to reverse these changes.

Aging is a physiological process that at times is only remotely connected to chronological age. One of my patients is a twenty-nine-year-old male. You've seen his sculptured physique in magazine advertisements and television commercials for everything from swimwear to cigarettes. To look at him is to see the picture of perfect health, achieved by at least four hours spent daily in the gym. But biologically he was on an advanced aging track. It was taking him longer to see results when he trained. He was increasingly tired and listless. He was becoming depressed. And he was getting muscle injuries, strained tendons and ligaments. Diagnostic tests revealed a hormonal imbalance and a loss of bone density, both signs of advanced aging. While he had masked his problems with a musculature finely tuned with extensive workouts, biologically he was ten to fifteen years older than his chronological age. A regimen of lifestyle change, diet, and supplements reversed his pro-aging condition.

Another way that biological aging differs from chronological aging is that it is not uniform. On your fortieth chronological birthday, your friends and family celebrate "all of you" reaching that societal milestone—not just, say, your arms and your lungs. But from a biological perspective, different parts of you age at different rates. In the scenario of normal healthy aging, your brain shrinks overall by about 6 percent from mature adulthood to advanced old age, but certain parts of it can shrink by as much 45 percent. In the digestive tract, the colon more or less functions the same at twenty-five as at sixty-five, but the kidneys and bladder begin showing pronounced signs of aging by fifty. Your sense of taste peaks at around age six, eyesight at ten, and bone density in the twenties. Dopamine and acetylcholine, two of the three major neurotransmitters—the brain's messengers that play a vital role in the aging process—rapidly decline with middle age, while the third, serotonin, usually remains at youthful levels.

On a cellular level, aging occurs every moment as old cells are not replaced by new ones. *Apoptosis,* or programmed cell death, is a normal part of any organism's life—with a few exceptions. Of those exceptions, two occur in the human body: cancer, which produces death, and sperm, which produces life. These cell types don't experience the programmed obsolescence of apoptosis, and for all intents and purposes are immortal, with the capacity to keep regenerating and replenishing their numbers.

The most dramatic examples of differences between chronologi-

cal age and biological age can be seen in sufferers of two "premature aging" diseases, progeria and Werner's syndrome. Patients with
these genetic diseases begin showing classic signs of advanced aging
in childhood or adolescence, including osteoporosis, graying and
thinning hair, wrinkled skin, a weakened cardiovascular system,
and an increased risk of diseases associated with the later years, including diabetes and cancer.

While the seeds of advanced aging can be sown at any age, generally speaking the most noticeable changes take place between the
ages of 40 and 50. Most physiological functions peak in the twenties, ride a plateau in the thirties, and begin to take a sharp descent
in the forties. Various internal biological mechanisms function in
synchrony until the onset of middle age when they begin their
downward march in lockstep. Canadian researchers Richard Earle
and David Imrie found that during this "decade of vulnerability"
the average North American male ages 15.2 years, while the average female ages 18.6 years.

The exact point at which the decline into advanced aging begins
is different for everybody. But without antiaging intervention—the
purpose of this book—here is what you can expect to happen to
your fifty-year-old body:

Brain: The brain shrinks 6 percent in size, resulting in a loss of cog-
    nitive abilities. Forgetfulness increases, and it is more difficult to
    process simultaneous streams of information. The decline is off-
    set somewhat by a greater accumulation of knowledge and ex-
    perience, which philosophers call wisdom.
Vision: Farsightedness among our aging baby boomer population
    made designer eyeglasses fashionable in the eighties. A loss of
    elasticity in the eye's lens makes it difficult to focus on nearby
    objects. Older eyes are also slower to adjust to darkness (as the
    pupils have a decreased capacity to dilate) from a loss of the
    rods—photoreceptors in the retina. Color perception starts to
    decline after you hit forty (especially for the yellow-blue color
    spectrum because the clear lens not only thickens but becomes
    more yellowish in color).
Hearing: While it is unusual for a fifty-year-old to wear a hearing
    aid, audiologists fear a tidal wave of advanced hearing impair-

ment among the baby boomers because of their predilection in earlier years for very loud music. Usually sensitivity to the higher tones is lost first.

Smell and Taste: These two senses are inextricably linked. Taste buds and olfactory receptors lose sensitivity, which is a primary reason that older people enjoy food less (and eat less). Zinc deficiency of the elderly also contributes to a diminution in taste. Pollution and smoking are two environmental factors thought to accelerate the aging of these senses.

Skin: How fast you wrinkle depends on a host of factors including genetics, nutrition, and environment. But the skin begins losing its elasticity in the twenties as collagen decreases. By fifty, thinning outer layers of skin cause it to sag. Sun damage and clumping of melanocyte (pigment) cells produce all kinds of brown blotches, the so-called liver spots, and abnormal growths.

Hair: Fifty percent of men have some balding by age fifty, and half of all men and women of European descent will have at least some gray hair. (The onset of graying appears a decade later in non-Europeans.)

Fat and Muscle: The ratio of muscle to fat begins its decline around thirty, with deposits of fat tissue peaking around fifty. More fat accumulates in and around the belly, buttocks, and thighs. The abdomen begins to sag because of lost muscle tone. Maximum grip strength drops from one hundred pounds at age thirty to about seventy-five pounds. While weight may stabilize at age fifty, the muscle-to-fat ratio continues to decrease well into the eighties.

Bones: Progressive loss of mineral content and density, notably calcium, results in increasingly brittle bones. The decline in women after the onset of menopause is about twice as fast as men. Not only are bones easier to break, but they are also harder to repair.

Urinary Tract: The kidneys begin to shrink in size and function at thirty, steadily losing the ability to remove waste products from the blood. The bladder, which collects the urine sent from the kidneys, loses its elasticity, which means less capacity and more trips to the bathroom.

Sex: Women experience menopause around fifty when their estrogen levels rapidly drop and ovulation ends. Men have a less pronounced sex hormonal decline, with testosterone concentrations diminishing gradually from the thirties. Intercourse for women can be painful as vaginal walls become thin and lubrication decreases. Sperm count in men dramatically decreases around fifty as tissues within the testes begin to thicken. It also takes about twice as much time to get an erection than at age twenty-five.

Heart: By age fifty the heart will have beat about 2 billion times. The heart muscle begins to enlarge to pump more blood to compensate for stiffening arteries. But the covering sheath around the heart thickens with age, leading to an overall decrease in output. This reduced output results in a decline in the supply of oxygen to muscle tissue, decreasing aerobic power and making it more tiring to climb stairs or walk up a hill.

Lungs: As lungs lose their elasticity, the capacity to breathe declines 20 percent by age fifty. Smokers, as you might guess, lose their lung function much earlier.

As we will learn in the next chapter, throughout recorded history mankind has valiantly resisted the advancement of age. The difference now is that we are the first of our species who can effectively intervene in the aging process.

ᨳ 3 ᨳ

Antiaging Medicine:
History and Theories

Humans have been thinking about aging for a long time. Gerontology, the science that deals with aging, is an invention of the late twentieth century, but theories about why we age and how possibly to halt it were in the minds of the ancients. The early Greeks, who weren't above using makeup to cover wrinkles and age spots—and we're talking about the men here—were the first to put thoughts on paper. They came up with the theory of the "four humors"—*humor* in the biological sense of the word, meaning any animal or plant fluid.

The Greek philosopher Empedocles (c. 490–430 B.C.) theorized that all of Nature was composed of four "root" elements: earth, wind, fire, and water. These four elements come together in various combinations to form all living things—a little more wind for a flower, a little more fire for an ox. From there it was an easy jump to theorize that the aging process itself is a disease that results from an imbalance of the four fluids in man that relate to the elements: blood, phlegm, yellow bile, and black bile.

Empedocles' concept was interesting in one other way that relates to antiaging medicine. He theorized that two different, opposing forces were at work in Nature. Rather romantically (at least from a jaded twentieth-century perspective) he called these two forces "love" and "strife." Love binds things together—plants, animals, Greek city-states—and strife separates them. Antiaging scientists would later adopt Empedocles' dichotomous forces for the theories of cellular entropy (disorder).

Now let's zoom across the history of antiaging medicine, passing centuries of alchemists, wizards, shamans, snake-oil salesmen, and adventurers who tried but failed to find an elixir of eternal life, tipping our hat along the way to Ponce de León who at least discovered Florida in the process. Arriving at the late nineteenth century, we find French physiologist Charles-Edouard Brown-Séquard promoting the extracts of crushed animal testicles as the fountain of youth. Although proven wrong, he is credited with suggesting hormonal-endocrine agents as an antiaging therapy.

The next significant news about aging occurs in the 1940s as scientists begin to theorize that genetic mutations are responsible for aging, that is, increasing mistakes made at the chromosome level cause widespread deterioration of the physiology. A couple of decades later, in 1961, anatomist Leonard Hayflick is called the father of modern antiaging research for his discovery of cellular aging. He proves that cells do not live eternally but rather have a finite life. After dividing about fifty times, cells suddenly stop, weaken, and die. And cells from older people die more quickly than cells from younger people in a laboratory. This gives rise to the notion of an "aging clock" that might be "reset" if only the clock could be found.

In the last thirty years, theories of aging have fallen in and out of fashion. In a recent paper presented to the Los Angeles Gerontology Research Group at the UCLA School of Medicine, Dr. L. Stephen Coles, M.D., Ph.D., identified twenty-five current theories of aging. A good example of how new research tends to make mincemeat of the best theories is the case of telomeres.

Telomeres are DNA sequences that cap and protect the ends of chromosomes. Geneticists noticed that each time a cell divided, its telomere became shorter. Could telomeres be the aging clock? Could stopping the telomeres from shortening halt the aging process? Could lengthening them restore youth? Heightening the drama, researchers in the 1980s discovered an enzyme that preserved telomeres; they dubbed it "telomerase." "The agent for eternal life had been found," gushed *Time* magazine. Unfortunately, subsequent findings revealed that telomeres do not always shorten significantly with age. Indeed, new research indicates that telomeres shrink and lengthen again and again over time.

As for the other twenty-four theories afloat, they can be classified into two schools: the school of chance and the school of grand design. The first school, which includes the classic "wear-and-tear" theory and "accumulation of trash" theory, points out that the human body with its 7 trillion cells is one incredibly complex bioenergy-producing machine. As with any manufacturing process, over time the body produces its share of trash and its biomechanisms begin to deteriorate. Chief among the toxic junk are free radicals, a by-product of energy metabolism, and advanced glycosylation end products (AGES), but there are also deformed enzymes, unrepaired DNA, and stress-damaged proteins. Chromosomes suffer wear and tear, and as the body's normal repair systems begin to falter, still more crud piles up. Which of these toxic by-product systems kills you first is a matter of chance, or it could be a matter of their collective ill will.

Free radicals are a story of good molecules gone bad. Inside all cells are little bean-shaped organisms called mitochondria that generate power for the cell, a process that produces excess electrons which, if left unattended, can do serious damage. But the body has concocted a way to mop up this waste—a natural antioxidant defense system. The air we breathe contains oxygen that, when mixed with the cell's fuel (mainly glucose) in the mitochondria, leads to energy production (similar to the combustion in your car engine) and waste product molecules (exhaust fumes) harboring errant electrons. When our antioxidant enzyme defense system is working correctly, it turns dangerous oxidation waste products into harmless water or other molecules. It is a brilliant defense mechanism but, alas, not perfect. Sometimes stray molecules with unpaired electrons (free radicals) beat the odds and sneak by the antioxidant cleanup crew. And the first thing they do is attach themselves to another molecule in the cell or in other cells. This extra electron destabilizes the former good citizen molecule, causing it to act with reckless abandon, ricocheting around the cell and other cells in the neighborhood and damaging everything in its path. And for various reasons the production of free radicals increases with age just as the body's natural antioxidants (free-radical fighters) decrease.

Glucose metabolism tends not to age very gracefully, either. The body's primary fuel source, glucose is a simple sugar produced by the breakdown of the carbohydrates we consume in the form of breads, pastas, fruits, and vegetables. As we age, excess glucose throughout the body binds to proteins, which are essential components in the ability of cells to repair and regenerate. Diabetes, a proaging disease that affects vital organs, is an extreme expression of what happens when excess glucose and insulin are out of balance.

The school of chance doesn't pretend to answer the questions of what and where the aging clock is. Rather, it asks why we should waste time trying to find the aging clock when we know what damages its mechanisms. Antioxidant supplements that immobilize free radicals and drugs that act as AGES solvents, including the new research medication pimagedine, are among some of the treatments devised to halt the aging process.

The school of grand design, on the other hand, is much neater. Death is not some messy, random biological event, but instead it is programmed into our cells. Find the (genetic) switch to the aging clock, and the aging process can be halted or even reversed. Despite or perhaps because of its exquisite simplicity, the school of grand design was beginning to fall out of favor for lack of definable results until the telomere theory came along. The quasi-debunking of telomeres as a cause of aging has been a big blow to the grand design school, but there are alternate master plan theories waiting in the wings. (See chapter 18 for new research on genetic causes of aging.)

Scientists believe that premature aging diseases such as progeria and Werner's syndrome may be caused by a single mutant gene, which may also be involved in the aging process in all humans. The completion of the Human Genome Project, which is mapping all of the about 100,000 human genes, should be completed before the year 2005 and is eagerly awaited by geneticists for the clues it might provide to aging. In the meantime, some students of the grand design school are focusing on results and looking for ways to use genetic reengineering to halt the aging process—in particular the body parts that age more quickly than others, such as the kidneys and the frontal cortex of the brain.

Which school of aging theories is right? Is aging a series of random events or a predetermined master plan that turns off human life around one hundred years? To some degree all twenty-plus theories and the two schools are correct. Aging appears to be a multi-level, overlapping process, and most scientists—with notable exceptions—reject the theory of a single cause of aging. Take, for example, DNA, the molecule in each cell that contains the fundamental genetic blueprint for the entire body. DNA figures prominently in many theories. AGES, those gooey masses of proteins and glucose, probably harm not only organs but also DNA, thus preventing cells from repairing themselves. Ah, then, that would indicate a genetic cause of aging. On the other hand, the genetic Holy Grail—a gene that turns the aging process on and off—might resemble less an instantaneous on-and-off switch than a gradual accumulation of junk that literally "gums up the works." Research indicates that there may be thousands of "trash" genes, nonproductive genes that are linked to disease and that accumulate in the gene pool, irreparably modifying DNA so that it programs cells to a limited life span.

Recently, there has been a movement to find common ground among the various theories, a biogerontological equivalent of physics' Grand Unified Theory. There seems to be little dispute, for example, that the human species was designed primarily to live long enough to sexually reproduce and raise the next generation. Twentieth-century humans have interrupted this orderly system of species preservation with their ability to contain infectious diseases. All parties agree that the human biological systems deteriorate over time, reaching a peak efficiency just after sexual maturation.

This type of change has been studied by physicists using the theories of thermodynamics, which attempt to explain the relationship between heat and energy. Briefly, it says no system can sustain a peak level of performance; deterioration is inevitable and builds on itself. Physicists call this increasing disorder "entropy." We'll discuss entropy and human aging in chapter 5, but for now it is sufficient to say that, like Empedocles' opposing elements of love and strife, the billions of cells that comprise the human body are constantly waging a battle between order and disorder. Death is the ultimate expression of disorder.

In the history of antiaging medicine, the most dramatic results in attempts to extend the life span have been achieved via an intervention many of us personally can relate to: caloric restriction. Many studies with laboratory animals show that when caloric intake is restricted by 30 percent, they live 30 percent longer. Why? It appears that restricting calories lowers the body temperature and slows down different parts of the metabolic system, that is, it slows cell division. In the process, less pro-aging free radicals are produced. A nutrient-rich, caloric-restrictive diet for humans *might* add an extra thirty years to the life span. But of course there are no guarantees and, so far, few human guinea pigs willing to spend a cold and hungry existence to prove a point.

Most of us are interested in extending the quality of life at a reasonable price rather than the quantity of life at any price. In the coming chapters we will see how advances in antiaging medicine for the first time in history are allowing us to achieve this goal.

4

The Critical Point
and the Theory of
Human Thermodynamics

From 1978 to 1996 the UCLA track and field team was the perfect laboratory for studying human physiology or, more precisely, how to fine-tune it. The pantheon of Olympic athletes who emerged from this program remains unparalleled: Flo-Jo Joyner, Steve Lewis, Gail Devers, Mike Powell, Jackie Joyner-Kersee, Willie Banks, and Kevin Young, among others. Each of them was a multiple gold medal winner or world record holder who advanced the boundaries of human athletic performance.

It was during my work as an attending physician at UCLA Sports Medicine and Rehabilitation Clinics, during track meets and training sessions at Drake Stadium and in the weight room, that I began seeing the parallels between these extraordinary athletes and my middle-age patients in private practice. After a while it became quite obvious that both sets of patients were on an advanced aging track.

The Critical Point

The elite athlete is constantly waging a battle against an enemy called *catabolism*. Essentially, catabolism is characterized by a breakdown of the body's physiological systems, the muscle and bone tissue being especially relevant to competitive athletes. When muscle and bone tissues are weakened, injuries increase, and enough injuries can end an athlete's career in a very short period of time. The opposite of this condition is *anabolism*, a state in which the body's systems are constantly replenishing themselves with new and stronger tissue growth.

Elite athletes and their coaches know there is a razor-thin line between training hard and overtraining. The exact point between the two conditions is what I call the "Critical Point." On one side of the Critical Point, the body is in an anabolic or rejuvenating mode. On the other side, it falls into a spiraling decline, a catabolic condition.

Elite athletes want to avoid a catabolic state. Unfortunately, it is unavoidable. Since a fraction of a second can often mean the difference between victory and defeat, world-class athletes are constantly pushing the envelope in their training until inevitably they cross over their Critical Point and throw their bodies into catabolic disrepair. This is when I would be brought in to restore their *anabolic drive capacity*—to readjust their physiologies to a regenerative mode.

I remember working with Steve Lewis, one of the best middle-distance runners ever. Winner of gold medals in the 400-meter and 400-meter-relay races in the 1988 Olympic Games, Steve, at the time of the 1992 Olympic Games, was headed down a catabolic path. He still managed to pick up a silver medal for the 400-meter, but clearly he was not at his peak performance. Shortly after he returned from the '92 Olympic Games in Barcelona, I gave him a complete physical and laboratory exam, and diagnosed the following:

◆ A depressed immune system: Steve was experiencing flu-like symptoms because a decline in his immune functions was making him susceptible to infectious agents such as viruses.

◆ Bell's palsy: This is a type of facial paralysis caused by viruses or by a decline or dysfunction in the body's nerve energetics—neurotransmission. As a result, the sufferer can look tired and depressed.

◆ Aches and pains: Steve's muscles were aching and his joints creaking. This was partially due to the viral infections, but his psychological profile also revealed that his serotonin neurotransmitter levels were low, which meant he was actually feeling more pain than he should have.

◆ Chronic fatigue: Steve was constantly lethargic. Where before he genuinely looked forward to the prospect of getting up each morning to train, he now found it hard to get out of bed. The energy and drive that helped him win two gold medals in the 1988 Olympic Games were gone.

◆ Sleep disorder: Even though Steve was tired, he could not get a good night's sleep. His sleep cycle was fragmented, characterized by frequent waking. He was missing stages of deep, nondream sleep when the body secretes two vital restorative hormones, growth hormone (anabolic) and melatonin (regulatory), which are vital for the immune and musculoskeletal systems.

Does the combination of these conditions sound familiar? They should if you have an elderly parent or relative. These are signs of aging. Aging and overtraining are physiologically very similar.

Human Thermodynamics

To repeat an oft-quoted analogy, elite athletes are like fine sports cars. Their highly tuned physiologies are the models to which the rest of us four-door sedans and station wagons compare ourselves. But there is one group of human beings that leaves the best of the elite athletes in the dust in terms of the efficiency of their physiological engines. Who are these hot-rodders? Children.

The average kid is a paragon of energy efficiency. I look at my own young daughters and see extremely sophisticated anabolic biomachines (that is, until the chocolate ice cream on their new clothes brings me back to earth). Their ability to generate and repair cells far surpasses any of the athletes at UCLA. Week to week, month to month, their bodies defy Carnot's theory of thermodynamics.

Thermodynamics is the science concerned with the relations between heat and energy. Nicolas-Léonard-Sadi Carnot was a French engineer whose interest was in making mechanical engines work more efficiently. While working on the efficiency of heat engines (that change heat energy into mechanical energy), he developed the Second Law of Thermodynamics, which states that closed physical systems if left alone will run down and become less organized. With the use of a different set of mathematical equations, he showed how the amount of disorder could be measured by determining its degree of *entropy*, that is, the amount of energy unavailable to perform work.

Entropy is the only known physical variable in Nature that mirrors the effects of time on a biological system. Unlike engines, humans *are* open systems. Our internal biochemistry and physiology constantly interact with the environment. We eat food, process and store some of it, and eliminate the rest. We inhale oxygen and exhale carbon dioxide. The computer science principle of "garbage in, garbage out" is not applicable to human machinery. But even accounting for this difference, our biological systems *do* follow the core of Carnot's tenet: Left alone, the human body will run down, become less biologically organized, increase its degree of entropy, and decrease its efficiency to build and repair vital systems. The greater the entropy, the greater the disorder or chaos.

Children, if left alone, will cause chaos of an entirely different kind, but biologically speaking, their bodies are in a super antientropic mode. Give them a little food (or, in the case of adolescent boys, a lot of food) and water, and their bodies pretty much take care of themselves. Indeed, they prosper. The rest of us, including elite athletes, need more help.

Our resting metabolic rate is the amount of heat our bodies produce at rest (that is, entropy). When we have an infectious illness with a high fever or a high stress level, we have excessive entropy (disorder), and for a very good reason: The body temporarily shuts down or decelerates various anabolic repair functions to focus on the problem at hand (such as an illness or a pack of rottweilers hot on our heels). Our biosystem is challenged by the cellular disorganization imposed by our perceptions of danger. Our response if appropriate and organized leads us back to the proper equilibrium and health.

When children are growing, they have a high resting metabolic rate (RMR); they defy the Second Law of Thermodynamics, at least for as long as they remain children. As we age there is less energy production and (normally) a lower metabolic rate. If the random events encountered in life (illness and those darn rottweilers) are not controlled either by our internal defenses or external intervention such as antibiotic therapy, then excess entropy leads to the ultimate degree of biological entropy disorder) known as death. With the use of antiaging therapy, our RMR can be increased by increasing the body's muscle mass. By increasing our muscle mass, our RMR automatically goes up. An increase of fat tissue decreases the RMR because fat, unlike muscle, is an inactive tissue. Like kids, we, too, can thumb our noses at Carnot's law of entropy.

Resetting the Critical Point

All of human life fits into a neat little "thermodynamic" triangle of (1) conception and childhood, (2) sexual maturation and reproduction, and (3) postreproduction and decline. During the development of an embryo there is the production of cellular organization. This is a state of antientropy, or *extropy*, which leads to the building of organized biological structures, the ultimate blueprint that calls for sexual maturation and reproduction.

After reproduction, the human organism stays in a state of bio-limbo for a while and then reaches a Critical Point where order turns to disorder, anabolism to catabolism, and regeneration to degeneration.

Athletes prematurely reach their Critical Point by overtraining, after which their athletic performance takes a nosedive and they experience the same symptoms as Steve Lewis: depressed immune system, chronic fatigue, aches and pains, and sleeplessness. Weakened muscle and bone tissue results in more injuries, which take longer to heal because of an elevated cortisol blood level and lowered testosterone and growth hormone concentrations, resulting in less training, weaker muscles and bones, and so on.

But we can bring the overtrained athlete out of his physiological tailspin. Through a program of supplements, diet, exercise, and lifestyle alterations, we can reset the body's control mechanisms.

We all have an automatic, built-in Critical Point, that moment when our bodies cannot maintain and repair our major physiological systems. The body switches from an essentially anabolic condition to one that is catabolic. This moment is not accompanied by trumpets, or, appropriately, violins, nor do we wake up one day and suddenly sag. We notice the changes gradually, but the Critical Point can be measured in middle-aged patients just as it can in elite athletes.

If we are not out to set a world record, when do we reach the

Critical Point? Generally speaking, we can expect to reach our Critical Point around the age of forty, give or take four or five years. With the onset of middle age, we begin to walk a tightrope between anabolic and catabolic states. A minor physical injury (such as a car accident), a psychological trauma (such as a divorce) or a lifestyle change (a job loss) causes stress that can upset the delicate balance and push us over the edge. We begin to head downward into a negative spiral, losing the capacity to repair our bodies. The end doesn't happen all at once, of course, but the descent has begun.

That's the bad news. Now here's the *good* news: The descent into catabolism is *not* inevitable. Our Critical Point *can* be reset in the same way elite athletes reset theirs. The threshold between anabolism and catabolism is different for all of us and depends on a number of factors ranging from genes to lifestyle choices. But with advances in antiaging medicine, we no longer have to sit on the sidelines and watch our best years race by. We can halt and even reverse many aspects of the aging process.

Signs of the Critical Point

Diagnostic tests have been developed over the last five years that can indicate whether you've reached your Critical Point (see sidebar, Pinpointing Your Critical Point). Here is what a doctor and a good scientific laboratory might see when examining a middle-aged patient or an overtrained athlete who is in catabolic decline:

1. Increased cortisol production: Cortisol, a hormone made by the adrenal gland, increases due to stress or overtraining. Left untreated, it can cause rising glucose levels and insulin insensitivity, which can result in an increase in fat mass and even diminished memory.
2. Decreased serum free testosterone (in both men and women): This results in a feeling of staleness and depression, and a decrease in lean tissue (bone and muscle) mass. Muscle definition is lost.
3. Decreased ratio between testosterone and DHEA levels and cortisol: DHEA (Dehydroepiandrosterone) is a natural hormone produced by the adrenal gland and has many different functions, from being a sex hormone precursor to having

neurological and immunological effects. As cortisol increases, testosterone and DHEA levels go down, resulting in weakness, feelings of stress, decreased coping mechanisms, emotional instability, poor sleep, and hypochondriacal complaints. Muscles are softer and have less tone and definition despite increased exercise.

4. Increased resting heart rate: The heart rate is elevated when it should not be, and the norepinephrine and epinephrine systems are turned on for no apparent reason. This is the "early phase" of the Critical Point. In the "late phase," the heart rate at rest may actually be lower because the catecholamine-alerting system has been depleted; it is shut down because it is worn out. This may indicate that your body is in a pronounced catabolic state.

5. Injuries: Muscle pulls, stress fractures, and tendinitis become more frequent. Cortisol dissolves tissues, which is why it is given by injection for conditions such as tennis elbow where excessive scar tissue is causing chronic pain and inflammation. Elite athletes are often given cortisone (cortisol) injections around the tendon under the kneecap for chronic pain or inflammation. I know of one unfortunate athlete who had several injections. One day he was doing some training involving jumps, and both kneecap tendons tore off. This is a classic example of cortisol excess leading to weakened tissue strength and injury. If you have ever had a cortisone injection, you may have noticed how the skin around the area became thinner. This is also why dermatologists tell you not to use strong steroid- or cortisone-based creams on the face.

6. Women: Loss of menstrual cycles and decreased estrogen. When the menses stops from excessive exercise, stress, weight loss, or fat loss, the protective effects of estrogen and progesterone are lost. The ability of bones to absorb minerals such as calcium decreases at the same time the intestines increase their absorption of these nutrients. Bone is a living and constantly changing tissue; it is continuously being laid down and remodeled as your activities and metabolism change. Some young but overtrained women athletes I have treated have had the fragile bones of postmenopausal women.

7. Excessive weight loss or weight gain: Weight loss initially oc-

curs during the first phase Critical Point when the catecholamine neurotransmitters increase, resulting in a loss of appetite. Later there is weight gain when the vegetative, lethargic phase of the Critical Point is reached as the serotonin neurotransmitter system begins to dominate. All the body's systems are dampened and slowed down with the weight.

8. Decreased growth hormone level: During acute stress, growth hormone (GH) increases, but as stress continues, GH and IGF-1 (a more stable blood measure of GH status) usually decrease. Decreased GH levels lower the ability to repair and rebuild tissues. With less GH released, body fat levels go up and energy levels go down.

9. Decline in immune function: Overtrained athletes catch colds and viruses more easily, and their illnesses last longer. Bursal cells, which make antibodies (infection-fighting proteins) decline. The blood levels of the important infection-fighting amino acid glutamine decline. Glutamine is important to the integrity and function of the lining of the intestinal tract for nutrient absorption as well as for healthy functioning of the brain and immune system.

Even without today's sophisticated biotechnology, there are telltale signs that you may be nearing your Critical Point:

Early signs

1. Vitality disappears. You no longer have a sense of well-being, confidence, and optimism. Your energy level is lower. You don't enjoy your life as much.
2. Declining libido. You lose interest in sex.
3. More aches and pains. You feel your body is falling apart.
4. Longer healing process. An injury—a cut, a pulled muscle— takes longer to heal.
5. Finger- and toenails grow at a slower rate.
6. You catch more colds and other infections more easily.

Late signs

1. Muscle loss. You become flabby as your fat mass is taking over.
2. Significant weight loss. Weight loss of 15–20 percent or more from your ideal body weight for no apparent reason can indicate a serious catabolic state.
3. Strange infections and recurrent fevers. As your immune system declines, infectious diseases that you were not susceptible to before suddenly rear their ugly heads. Shingles, Bell's palsy, cytomegaloviruses, herpes and Epstein Barr viruses may take up residence in your body. You experience frequent unexplainable flu-like symptoms from recurrent viral or other infectious reactivation, or your own immune system goes haywire and attacks your own tissues.
4. Depression. You are gripped by a sense of hopelessness and doom. The ultimate catabolic stage, death, no longer seems distant or unwelcome.

Just as your Critical Point is individual and unique, *how* to reset it is also specific to your physiology. If only I could treat every athlete or middle-aged patient the same way, my work would be easy. But therapy for Steve Lewis would not work for Gail Devers, who, like Lewis, suffered a decline in athletic performance between the 1988 and 1992 Olympic Games. In Steve's case, his treatment involved a regimen to boost his immune system and correct his chronic fatigue. Gail's regimen, on the other hand, focused on treating one particular hormone imbalance. Once correctly diagnosed and treated, Gail quickly turned her career around. In 1988 she went home empty from the games at Seoul. Four years later, after she received proper therapy, I was privileged to witness her gold medal–winning performance in the 100-meter race at the Barcelona games.

This book is unlike other books on antiaging because it shows you how to build a personal antiaging regimen that is right for you. We all have different Critical Points, and *how* we age is also different. One catchall antiaging program cannot work. In the next two chapters you'll learn more about the importance of hormones and neurotransmitters in the aging process. But if you're anxious to begin creating your Personal Antiaging Regimen, you can start immediately by skipping to chapter 7.

Pinpointing Your Critical Point

There are a number of high-tech tests you can take to further assess your Critical Point. None of these is necessary to complete your Personal Antiaging Regimen, but they provide additional insight into exactly how quickly you are aging. Many of these tests are used to analyze the overtraining of elite athletes. These tests must be ordered by your doctor.

Muscle/Protein Catabolism Tests

In a catabolic decline, your body loses protein and muscle mass, resulting in increased protein oxidation. Two tests can measure this loss:

1. Have your health professional run a routine blood chemistry panel, which contains a number for your blood urea nitrogen (BUN) level. The BUN number can be a marker of protein breakdown by oxidation or the elimination of urea by your kidneys. Either one can indicate an early protein problem. If the number is very low, it may mean an inadequate protein intake. A high-normal value can mean a pronounced breakdown of protein (if kidney function is normal), or be a marker of excessive protein intake. The BUN number has no significance unless you track it over time and correlate it with your exercise level and protein intake. It is a rough guide about the status of the breakdown and elimination of proteins in your body. If the BUN rises abnormally because your kidneys cannot eliminate it, this can indicate serious kidney malfunction or even failure, or a liver problem.
2. The loss of lean mass and its replacement by fat can be measured by using a caliper, by an electrical impedance device, or by an underwater weighing test for body composition.

Lowered Blood Albumin Levels Tests

If you have had a general chemistry panel conducted in the last few years, compare your previous levels of blood albumin, a protein, with your current level. A declining serum albumin is associated with decreased longevity. You may be getting closer to your Critical Point when your body cannot maintain an adequate blood albumin level.

Increased Entropy Test

You and your doctor can obtain at-home salivary kits that determine abnormal ratios and imbalances of the major hormone levels, including testosterone, estrogen, progesterone, DHEA, melatonin, and cortisol. These easy-to-use tests are available from several manufacturers. (See the Diagnostic Laboratories list in the appendix.) A catabolic condition may be indicated if the tests show increased cortisol levels throughout the whole day or abnormal peaks with corresponding decreases of testosterone and DHEA. Drastically decreased melatonin, progesterone, and estrogen levels also could indicate an approaching Critical Point.

Oxidative Stress Damage Test

Free radicals damage various cell components, including the genetic material known as DNA, the cell power generator known as mitochondria, and the cell membrane known as the lipid envelope. They also attack fat in the blood called LDL (low-density lipids), which when damaged become toxic to the blood vessel walls and cause inflammatory clogging of the arteries. The oxidative stress test measures the damage caused by free radicals.

Pro-oxidation State Test

Your rate of free radicals production can be measured by different chemical reactions in your body. Levels of metals, including iron and copper, and heavy metals (cadmium, lead, mercury, etc.) are determined to see how much they promote free radical generation.

Antioxidant State Test

What is your capacity to deal with free radicals? Tests can measure your antioxidant protection by your fat-soluble and water-soluble levels. The fat-soluble antioxidants are the carotenoid group (widespread group of naturally occurring pigments), the vitamin E family, CoQ10, and others. Vitamin C is the primary water-soluble antioxidant.

Repair of Oxidative Damage Test

What is your capacity to repair damaged components of your cells? (Ask your doctor about tests numbered 6, 7, 8, and 9 from the Genox Corp. of Baltimore, Maryland. See Diagnostic Laboratories in the appendix for more information.)

Glycation Index Test

How much has your blood sugar "caramelized" or linked up with the proteins of your body? Some scientists feel that the degree of glycation is a very strong indicator of your biological aging. A GlucoProtein (fructosamine) test measures the amount of glucose that is bound to your serum protein. A lower glycation number can indicate a lower aging rate. An increasing value can indicate an increased glycation/caramelization effect, a pro-aging factor. One test every three weeks can give you an idea about the direction of your caramelization factor and aging.

Vitamin and Mineral Absorption Tests

How well are you able to absorb vitamins and minerals into your serum and red blood cells? Having an adequate level of manganese and zinc, for example, is important to the production of antioxidant enzyme systems. If your ability to absorb vitamins and minerals is weak, your anabolic repair process declines. (See Diagnostic Laboratories in the appendix.)

Leaky Gut Detoxification Test

How well is your gut (digestive tract) working? Is it leaking? How good is your liver at detoxifying foreign and normally occurring substances? Tests are available to determine the permeability of your gut as well as the functionality of your detox systems—liver, kidneys, bowels. (See Diagnostic Laboratories in the appendix.)

Intestinal Flora Function Test (Dysbiosis Index)

What is the ratio between friendly and unfriendly bacteria in your intestines? Too much of the latter could cause immune dysfunction, poor digestion, memory problems, and weakness and fatigue. An abnormality is indicated by the Dysbiosis Index. (See Diagnostic Laboratories in the appendix.)

Immune Function Test

How good is your ability to fight infections? There are several discrete measures of the body's immune function, including tests for Natural Killer Cells, lymphocyte subsets (CD4, CD8 and others), and antibodies.

Testing Yourself at Home

These tests can be done at home without a doctor's prescription. If you respond "yes" to any of the following, this could indicate a catabolic condition.

- ◆ Triceps pinch: Pinch your triceps (the muscle on the back of the upper arm). Do you notice more flab than muscle there than ever before (without a loss of weight)?
- ◆ Skin: Is your skin thinner? (See chapter 14 for a skin elasticity test.)
- ◆ Heart rate: Measure your heart rate by putting your index and middle finger together and placing it over the artery next to your wrist, below the thumb, and feel your heartbeat. Take a one-minute count upon waking and measure it periodically over the next month or so. Keep a log and look at the general

trend. What is the direction? For women there will be fluctuations related to hormonal changes during the monthly menstrual cycle, so always measure on the same day of your cycle. It is important to establish a baseline while you feel in good health and are not on any medication or under abnormal stress. This is your "good health basal rate," and an unusual deviation from it can be cause for concern.

◆ Urine temperature: Urinate into a foam cup (foam to avoid cooling of the urine) when you first get up in the morning at least every other day for two weeks while feeling well and not under stress or using any medication. Check the temperature with an ovulatory type of thermometer that you can buy in a drugstore. This is your baseline "good health basal temperature." Repeat the test in two or more weeks, or sooner if you are not feeling well. Compare it to your "good health basal temperature." If the temperature is going down, it could indicate a lower metabolic rate and perhaps the need for thyroid hormone. If it is going up, you may be under infectious or inflammatory stress, have hormonal imbalances, or be experiencing acute psychological stress.

◆ GlucoProtein (fructosamine): This procedure is virtually identical to the procedure used for most self-tests for blood glucose. A fingerstick blood sample is placed on a test strip, and in four minutes the results are shown on a meter display.

5

The Magic Bullet: Hormonal Harmony and the Growth Hormone Family

It was the day before an important game for the UCLA Bruins basketball team that would determine who was the Pac 10 Conference leader. During practice the team's hotshot forward Reggie Miller, now with the National Basketball Association's Indiana Pacers, fell and had trouble walking off the court. My examination confirmed everybody's worst suspicions: a sprained ankle. I had no choice but to recommend that he sit out the next game. But Reggie was stubborn. "Uh-uh. Sorry, Doc. Tomorrow's game is too important. If I can walk onto the court, then I'm playing," he told me. I was adamant—he could not play. He was *more* adamant—he *was* going to play. And play he did. By the next day he had recovered enough from his sprain to put in, if not his best, a still outstanding performance that helped the Bruins to victory.

Reggie's athletic performance defied conventional medical wisdom. How did he do it? His body was in complete hormonal harmony.

In the last chapter we learned about *anabolic drive,* or the body's ability to repair itself. Anabolic drive is derived from the energy produced by the mitochondria, the power generators in your cells. At twenty-one years of age, Reggie was at his peak physical condition. His anabolic drive was near perfect. But he would not have played the game that day if his anabolic *capacity* had not also been at its maximum. Anabolic capacity is created when energy (fuel metabolized from glucose, fatty acids, and amino acids) is combined with the proper balance of hormones to make high-energy compounds, which then are used for muscle contraction, cell repair, and other functions.

The relationship between anabolic drive and anabolic capacity is mutually dependent. The cell's mitochondria power generators might be in top shape (anabolic drive), but they're not going anywhere without an adequate fuel and hormone supply (anabolic capacity). Similarly, your cells can have an adequate fuel/hormone supply (anabolic capacity) but can utilize only a minimum amount if their power generators (anabolic drivers) are in disrepair. Anabolic drive and anabolic capacity are at their maximum level when the body's hormones are in balance and at their peak levels. If you want to be physiologically youthful, then your body's hormones must be at youthful levels.

> **Anabolic Capacity**
> (fuel such as glucose)
>
> +
>
> **Anabolic Regulatory Hormones**
> (growth hormone, testosterone, insulin, thyroid)
>
> =
>
> **Anabolic Drive**
> (cell regeneration)

What exactly are hormones? They are molecular messengers of the neuroendocrine system, one of the body's four main biological systems. Think of hormones as the general command substances used by the body to regulate itself. Hormones are located in glands, including the liver, adrenal glands, hypothalamus in the brain, and pancreas. The brain signals the glands by using chemical messengers called neurotransmitters that are carried instantaneously from one nerve to another. We'll see in the coming chapters how neurotransmitters are vital components of the way we age and why we age differently from one another.

Hormones undergo a radical decline with aging. For most people, hormones peak in their twenties, stabilize for another decade or so, and then begin a steep decline. By age seventy, most of us will have less than 50 percent of the vital hormones we had in our youth. For example, growth hormone supplies are at 15 percent to 20 percent of peak levels by the time we are sixty or seventy.

The impact of declining hormones on the human body is irrefutable. Massive amounts of research have shown that declining hormones contribute to every aspect of aging, including loss of muscle, fragile bones, thinning skin, decreasing vision, increased heart attacks and strokes, and even a decrease in our sense of well-being. The value of replenishing hormones has been accepted for decades and is widely used today. Indeed, Premarin, the synthetic version of the female sex hormone estrogen, is the most widely pre-scribed prescription drug in America. Interestingly, the same logic that has prompted the medical establishment for decades to pro-mote the use of estrogen hormonal replacement therapy (as a safe and effective means of dealing with one particular aspect of aging, menopause) for some reason does not extend to the other hor-mones. But what is true for estrogen is true for the other hormones. To reverse the effects of aging, hormone supplies depleted by aging must be replenished.

Hormonal replacement therapy is an exquisitely simple concept that is somewhat complicated by the aging process itself. Some sci-entists have used the fact that hormone levels decline with aging to advocate an antiaging strategy of unrestricted hormonal replace-ment. They argue that reversing the debilitating effects of aging is as easy as restoring hormones to levels when you were at your peak at about twenty-eight. That sounds good on paper, but it doesn't work in reality. It is foolish to push the hormonal system of a fifty-year-old man or woman, for example, to peak levels without taking into account how the rest of the body has aged. The number of hormonal cell receptors also decline radically with aging. Flooding the body with excessive amounts of hormones is, at the very least, futile and wasteful, and, at worst, damaging and catabolic (pro-aging). Too high doses of hormones can speed up the body's machinery to the point where it begins to burn itself out. The hormones must also be balanced in relation to one another. One hormone out of balance with the others will throw the whole body out of whack.

The most effective way of dealing with diminished hormones is to make the body more sensitive to what is left. One strategy targets each individual hormone. For example, exercise and diet manage-ment can shrink fat cells, which makes them more receptive to insulin. Another strategy is to stimulate the supply of growth hor-mone, which we'll learn later is unique among the hormones be-cause of its allover renewing effect on the body.

We can fine-tune our hormonal systems to achieve proper harmony even as the body hormones naturally decline with aging. Changes associated with the aging process can be reversed through an *integrated* approach of appropriate hormonal replacement combined with manipulating diet, exercise, lifestyle, and various natural anabolic supplements.

The Seven Hormones

From an antiaging viewpoint, life after twenty-five is a battle to maintain order while time pushes you constantly toward greater disorder or greater entropy. I came up with the antiaging concepts of anabolic drive and capacity from my years of observing the world's best athletes push themselves into entropy—in other words, a temporary state of advanced aging—in order to reach the next level of athletic performance. As I tracked these athletes, I saw world records being broken in front of my eyes. How did these athletes maintain anabolic drive and capacity in the face of their grueling training? Can these principles be applied to an aging population and reverse some of the conditions associated with aging?

These elite athletes did remarkable and, yes, highly unconventional things to increase their performance—to run faster, jump higher, and throw a discus or javelin farther. They took injections of insulin even though they were not diabetic. They tried growth hormone, which previously had been used only for children with dwarfism. They ingested massive doses of vitamin pills even though they were not nutrient deficient. And they experimented with everything from amino acids to deer antler concoctions and other, even more exotic substances picked up along the Olympic grapevine from their counterparts in the former Soviet Union. The problem with most research on the effects of human aging is that it usually isn't done with human subjects. Experimenting with human volunteers is either very difficult (the problem of finding willing volunteers) or illegal because of restrictions imposed by the Federal Drug Administration and other regulatory bodies. So scientists use lab animals (usually mice or rats) to draw conclusions—which presents obvious problems. The elite athletes used themselves as guinea pigs. As they were increasing their athletic performance, they were also advancing antiaging therapy quite literally by leaps and bounds.

What did I learn from observing these athletes? That your anabolic drive and capacity are governed by a network of seven key hormonal systems that can be broken down into three groups:

1. The anabolic system, consisting of insulin, testosterone, and growth hormone.
2. The regulator system, notably the thyroid hormone.
3. The catabolic system, consisting of cortisol, glucagon, and the catecholamines (epinephrine and norepinephrine hormones).

Each of these key hormonal systems plays an important role in the aging process.

The Anabolic System

INSULIN: Insulin is an anabolic agent that everyone needs for energy storage and protein synthesis. When insulin is working properly, it promotes the synthesis and storage of glucose (needed for short-term energy) and fat (for long-term energy), and increases the formation of proteins, the body's building blocks, from amino acids. Insulin works as a transporter of glucose by binding it to receptors located on the surface of cells. When there isn't enough insulin, as in juvenile diabetes, you become thin and wasted because the cells don't receive sufficient glucose. The relationship of insulin to the adult form of diabetes is less clear cut. When there's too much insulin, the insulin receptors and insulin itself stop working properly. The body compensates by storing its basic fuel (glucose) where it will last the longest, in the fat cells, instead of distributing it between fat and muscle tissue, resulting in a weight gain.

TESTOSTERONE: This hormone has a wide range of physical and psychological effects on men *and* women. It initiates protein synthesis and skeletal muscle growth, increases bone density and red blood cell mass, and can increase strength when used in appropriately high doses. It can increase motivation and drive, and alleviates depression if levels are subnormal. It promotes growth hormone release and increases the metabolic rate, which burns fat.

GROWTH HORMONE: Released by the pituitary gland in spurts during deep sleep, growth hormone (GH) is unique in the anabolic system because it can alter the direction of many age-related changes. Among the well-known attributes of GH replacement are increased muscle and bone mass, decrease of body fat, strengthening of the immune systems, and generally promoting energy and a sense of well-being.

The Regulator System

The *thyroid hormone* is particularly sensitive to imbalance. Either too much or too little can result in pro-aging, catabolic effects. It has seven main activities:

1. Increases the body's oxygen consumption and heat production by stimulating all the tissues except the brain, spleen, and testes. It also regulates your resting metabolic rate (RMR). Taking too much can increase metabolism to a pro-oxidative, pro-aging condition. It also leads to osteoporosis. Having too little can lead to dementia, depression, and inertia.
2. Regulates the heart's rhythm and rate. Too much or too little can cause an irregular heartbeat.
3. Amplifies the effect of the catecholamine hormones. Too much can make you agitated and jumpy. Too little can make you unresponsive.
4. Regulates the body's waste disposal system. Too much can result in diarrhea and weight loss. Too little can result in constipation and weight gain.
5. Affects the neuromuscular system. Too much can increase deep tendon reflexes. Too little makes the nervous system sluggish and unresponsive. The right amount stimulates protein synthesis.
6. Regulates glucose and cholesterol levels. Too much can worsen diabetes. Too little elevates cholesterol, which can clog arteries.

7. Affects cortisol. Too much or too little can make cortisol act as a catabolic agent.

The Catabolic System

CORTISOL: Secreted by the adrenal gland, cortisol in the proper amount plays a vital emergency response function. In situations of extreme stress or danger, cortisol takes control of the neuroendocrine and metabolic networks, redirecting resources to the muscles and the brain's cognitive functions. In the movie "Mission Impossible" you can bet Tom Cruise's character's adrenals were pumping out cortisol like crazy as he held on to the train by his fingers. Cortisol becomes a problem when what is normally a temporary excess production becomes permanent, a condition of aging or chronic stress. In excess, it increases blood sugar, catabolizes muscle tissue, breaks down fat, and increases insulin levels, which results in more muscle wasting, bone loss, weight gain, abnormal fat distribution, decreased immune function, brain damage at the hippocampus, thinning of the skin, ulcers, increased blood pressure, and, in general, havoc with the thyroid and gonadal functions.

GLUCAGON: Like insulin, glucagon is concerned with energy and, as its name implies, particularly in processing glucose, which is metabolized from carbohydrates and is the primary source of fuel for all animals. The ratio between insulin and glucagon determines whether there is storage or depletion of energy stores. By releasing glucose from glycogen stores, glucagon makes energy available between meals. It also stimulates the liver to make glucose from amino acids and breaks down fat stores in the liver. Glucagon increases with age, which is bad because it promotes pro-aging by aggravating an already abnormal glucose metabolism and elevated glucose levels often present in the scenario of aging.

CATECHOLAMINES (EPINEPHRINE AND NOREPINEPHRINE): These work along with cortisol to provide the body with quick action in times of danger, stimulating the nervous system, increasing heart rate, expanding your ability to expend energy and generally making you more alert. Too much catecholamines can produce anxiety attacks and, if prolonged, can upset the insulin/glucagon ratio and promote aging.

Building an Anabolic Program

Building an effective antiaging program means rebalancing the hormonal system in favor of the anabolic system, that is, increasing the cells' anabolic drive (via the energy factories) and its anabolic capacity (fuel and hormone supply). A dual approach is needed to remove those factors that interfere with anabolic action and to promote those factors that stimulate anabolic action.

Remove Pro-Aging Factors

You must remove both the internal and external catabolic (pro-aging) factors from your life and environment. They cause chronic stress, which elevates cortisol levels. Eliminate factors that lower testosterone levels, including alcohol abuse (more than two drinks daily), use of illicit drugs (such as cocaine, marijuana, and amphetamines), inadequate rest, poor nutrition, and even excessive air travel. Certain medications also interfere with the release of testosterone and insulin, including cortisone tablets or injections and beta-blockers (such as propranolol and thiazides). Consult with your health care professional about alternatives to these medications. For more tips on removing catabolic factors from your life and environment, see chapter 13.

A proactive, antiaging program also promotes the anabolic hormones by increasing testosterone and growth hormone, and improving the functioning of insulin. Diet, exercise, and supplements all play a part.

An Anabolic Diet

An anabolic diet is high in protein. The rule of thumb for your *daily* protein requirement is $^1/_3$ gram of protein per pound of body weight for ordinary daily activities, $^1/_2$ gram for moderate exercise training, and $^3/_4$ to 1 gram for intensive tissue-building training. Generally speaking, it's a good idea to eat six meals of low to medium caloric content that are nutrient-dense instead of the traditional three or four large meals. Your diet must take into account your particular aging pathway (see chapter 7) and glucose metabolism track (see chapter 10).

Anabolic Exercise

For most of us, exercise is a semirandom program undertaken for the sake of general health. It is good for us (we think), but we don't know why. But a training program is a strategy with a specific goal—to build stronger legs, to run a 5K race faster, to improve a tennis backhand.

Athletes don't exercise, they train. They don't have time to waste on random exercise. An anabolic exercise—or, rather, training program—has a specific goal: to stimulate the release of testosterone and growth hormone. It concentrates on weight-resistance exercises for twenty to forty minutes, working the major muscle groups in two to three sets of six to eight repetitions. The effort should be intense. Consult a knowledgeable trainer before jumping into a program by yourself. (You will learn more about building an exercise program that fits into your aging pathway in chapters 7 through 10.)

Other anabolic exercises include bicycle sprints, running sprints, and other brief exercises that get you winded. Avoid prolonged and exhaustive exercises that can lower testosterone and growth hormone, such as marathon runs and triathlons. And avoid the "Weekend Warrior Syndrome" where all of your exercise is crammed into two days. That's a recipe for overtraining and injuries.

An anabolic training program has a dual benefit: increasing anabolic hormone levels while at the same time strengthening bones and muscles, making you more mobile and less prone to injury. Best of all, it's *never* too late to reap the rewards of an anabolic training program.

A recent study of one hundred nursing home residents reported in the *Journal of the American Medical Association* found that ten weeks of weight lifting doubled muscle strength in the legs, improved walking ability and increased the daily physical activity of subjects by about 35 percent. If residents of a nursing home can do it, what's stopping you?

Anabolic Supplements

Anabolic supplements build anabolic drive and capacity. If you begin an anabolic exercise program, consider taking the following supplements. (You will learn more about antiaging supplements in chapters 7 to 10.)

SOY-WHEY PROTEIN: Among the most efficient builders of anabolic capacity is soy-whey, a combination of soy protein extracts and whey. It is the natural by-product of milk, the stuff left over when cheese or homogenized milk is made. Soy-whey protein has a higher amount of the branch chain amino acids (leucine, isoleucine, and valine), which are more resistant to breakdown during exercise or stress. It also has a low glycemic index, which means there is less insulin stimulation and less fat storage potential. Soy-whey protein is usually sold as a powder to be mixed with water, fruit juice, milk, or soy milk. It is readily available at health and natural food stores. A lactose-free brand with no artificial sweeteners is your best choice.

The best time to use soy-whey protein is when your muscles are the most receptive to their amino acids—the organic substances that connect together to form proteins, the basic building blocks of muscle and other cells. This window of opportunity occurs within two hours after a workout when your growth hormone and testosterone levels are at their peak.

HIGH-GLYCEMIC FOOD: In the middle of your workout, eat a little high-glycemic food such as French bread or puffed rice crackers to stimulate the release of insulin; insulin moves amino acids into cells as part of its storage function. (See chapter 17 for a list of high-glycemic foods and beverages.) Do not use fructose fruit drinks because they are not potent insulin releasers; they have a lower glycemic index.

ANTIOXIDANTS: Antioxidants are not anabolic per se but help to decrease the damage to tissues from the catabolic effect of workouts. Increase your antioxidant intake when you increase the frequency, duration, or intensity of your exercise regimen. (See chapter 7 for more information about antioxidants.)

MITOCHONDRIAL PROTECTORS: Several anabolic supplements work directly to support the mitochondria, the cell's energy factories responsible for anabolic drive. These include CoQ10, alpha lipoic acid, acetyl L-carnitine, L-carnitine, natural Vitamin E and creatine monohydrate.

♦ Creatine Monohydrate (CM): Gives quick energy for a workout and helps in the most critical postworkout or recovery phase (when the muscle tissue is actually built).
♦ Acetyl L-carnitine: In addition to helping build mitochondria, it may also stimulate the production of testosterone.

OTHER SUPPLEMENTS: These supplements, which facilitate the anabolic process, are worth considering:

♦ Chromium and Vanadium: Enhance the action of insulin, thereby creating an anabolic effect.
♦ DHEA: Can increase testosterone and GH levels in postmenopausal women and some men (but not all). See chapter 14 regarding the pros and cons of DHEA. When using a pro-hormone like DHEA, keep in mind that it can have the opposite effect, that is, create more estrogen instead of testosterone.
♦ Boron: Promoted as a testosterone stimulator, but it has not been proven to be effective by healthy athletes. It may benefit menopausal women by enhancing estrogen.
♦ Omega-3 fatty acids: Fish oils rich in eicosapentaenoic (EPA) and decosahexaenoic acid (DHA) increase anabolic capacity by helping the immune system, blood clotting, and fat burning. Flax oil is another source of Omega 3s. (See chapters 7 and 11 for more information on smart oils.)
♦ Androstenedione and 4-Androstenediol: These natural hormones boost testosterone. Available over the counter, these potent supplements should be used under the supervision of a health-care specialist.
♦ L-Glutamine: This anticatabolic amino acid boosts levels of the important antioxidant called glutathione.
♦ N-Acetyl-Cysteine: This amino acid provides the building blocks to make glutathione.
♦ Magnesium: This mineral activates glucose utilization by cells, thereby producing an anabolic effect.

If you are already on a training program, you may have heard about so-called plant anabolic steroid agents that promise to build muscle mass. Examples are sarsaparilla, saw palmetto, beta-sitosterol, yohimbine bark extracts, and ecdysterone. Don't waste your money. They have no known anabolic effect and won't help build muscle tissue.

Anabolic Reserve

The body at any age holds in reserve an untapped amount of anabolic drive and capacity. The reversal from a pro-aging catabolic to an antiaging anabolic lifestyle can happen in a matter of months.

I am reminded of the second time I worked with Flo-Jo Joyner, the great track and field star. After an illustrious string of achievements as a college athlete, Flo-Jo by 1985 thought her career was over and had retired to work as a bank teller. When I saw her again at the UCLA Pauley Pavilion Sports Clinic, she was flabby and out of shape. But her coach, Bobby Kersee, had a dream of her making the U.S. Olympic team for the 1988 games in Seoul. In a little over two years, she not only made the team but went on to become the fastest woman in the world, setting world records in the 100-meter and 200-meter races and winning three gold medals at the Seoul games.

The lesson here is that an integrated and natural anabolic regimen of diet, training, and nutritional supplements can turn your life around. Your current physical condition and age are factors, not limitations. By the time you finish this book, you will have the tools to do things you never dreamed possible.

Growth Hormone Family: The Magic Bullet?

The rejuvenating effects of the naturally occurring anabolic hormone in the body known as growth hormone (GH) are just now coming to the attention of the public. In comparison to GH, DHEA and melatonin—two other hormones that have been the subject of dozens of articles and books—are relatively minor players in aging. Taken alone, GH's impact on an aging program is limited, as is the case with melatonin, DHEA, or any other substance. But as part of an integrated strategy, GH and its related compounds (see sidebar) are potent antiaging tools.

The Growth Hormone Family

Emerging science shows that there is more than one player in the overall physiology of growth hormone. An interplay of a group of compounds is now believed to be responsible for what previously was thought to be the sole domain of GH. Thus, "the magic bullet" is now believed to be a more sophisticated process involving various combinations of the following:

- ◆ Growth Hormone (GH)
- ◆ Insulin Growth Factor 1 (IGF-1)
- ◆ Growth Hormone Releasing Hormone (GHRH)
- ◆ Hexeralin
- ◆ Growth Hormone Releasing Peptide 2, third generation (GHRP-2)
- ◆ Non-Peptidal Oral Secretagogues (MKO677 and others)

Please note: These are pharmaceutical substances prescribed only under medical supervision. Supplements being offered directly to the consumer which tout pro-growth hormone effects are, essentially, ineffective and a waste of money. For example, some supposedly pro-GH supplements are sold in sublingual (under the tongue) tablets, spray, or fizzy tablets. In reality, GH and its family at this time can only be administered effectively through injection, except for MKO677, which is taken orally.

New Precautions

Growth hormone stimulates the production of a related compound called Insulin Growth Factor 1, produced in the liver, which serves as a marker for GH effect. (IGF-1 also independently stimulates growth.) Previously, it was thought the ideal was to raise IGF-1 to youthful levels (350 nanograms per milliliter or more). New research shows that a link exists between prostate cancer and high levels of IGF-1: in general, the higher the level of IGF-1, the higher the risk. However, the risk level dramatically increases when the level is over 185 ng/ml. Until further research is conducted, it is best to stay in a safe range of IGF-1.

Until the 1980s, the medical establishment viewed growth hormone (GH) as a physiological oddity, a throwaway, the hormonal equivalent of tonsils. It was known that GH was important for the growth of the skeletal system during childhood and adolescence; children who did not have enough GH were very short. Further research into GH was limited because the only source of GH was human cadavers. The little that was generated from this source went to children whose growth was abnormal.

In 1985 the first GH was synthesized; it was artificially made in laboratories using gene-splicing and cloning technologies. For the first time a relatively large and safe supply became available. The first hint of the potential of GH as an antiaging therapy came from European researchers who were following patients who had lost their pituitary glands from surgery and disease. When given GH, these patients unexpectedly showed a remarkable improvement in muscle and bone mass and psychological well-being.

In the United States in 1990, a team led by the late Daniel Rudman, M.D., conducted the first scientific GH study on a group of healthy men aged sixty-one to eighty; they were given a daily dose for six months. They found that the men gained muscle, lost fat, and developed thicker, more supple skin. "The magnitude of changes," said Dr. Rudman, was the equivalent of reversing "ten to twenty years of aging."

Many studies later, the list of benefits of GH replacement therapy as reported in the scientific literature continues to grow:

- ◆ increase in bone mineral content and density
- ◆ improved cardiac function/output
- ◆ improved kidney excretion capacity
- ◆ improved immune function
- ◆ better cholesterol, HDL, and LDL levels
- ◆ increased ability to exercise
- ◆ increased sense of well-being and energy
- ◆ decreased depression and irritability
- ◆ increased muscle mass and lowered body fat
- ◆ improved sexual pleasure and function

◆ restoration of heart, liver, spleen, kidneys, and other organs that shrink with age
◆ better vision
◆ deeper sleep
◆ younger-looking skin (improved elasticity and fewer wrinkles)
◆ hair growth

The above effects typically occur after six to twelve months of continued therapy. It was not until six years after Dr. Rudman's seminal study that the FDA officially approved the use and marketing of GH for adults deficient in the hormone. For the first time, in late 1996, pharmaceutical manufacturers made GH available to physicians for their adult patients.

Recent research has shown that GH and its family of compounds can take very ill patients out of heart failure, and studies are under way on treating neurodegenerative disorders such as amyotrophic lateral sclerosis (ALS, or Lou Gehrig's disease) and Alzheimer's. In my practice I have successfully treated patients with chronic fatigue, fibromyalgia, sciatica, pre-diabetic conditions, mental disturbances such as excessive irritability and depression, poor sleep, muscle weakness, and sexual dysfunctions.

Signs of Growth Hormone Deficiency

Growth hormone declines in middle age, so by the time you are sixty, you will have only a fraction of your peak level. When should you consider GH replacement therapy? There are a number of tests that can screen for GH deficiency, including the IGF-1 (Somatomedin C) blood test and the clonidine GH stimulation test. The GH-deficient adult usually shows many of these symptoms:

◆ reduced energy and vitality
◆ impaired emotional reactions
◆ social isolation
◆ low self-esteem
◆ emotional distress
◆ poor general health
◆ history of pituitary disease

- increased fat mass, especially around the belly
- decreased muscle mass, with reduced muscle tone and strength
- reduced exercise capacity
- dehydration
- reduced mineral density of bone (which increases bone fracture potential)
- reduced kidney function capacity (resulting in reduced urinary excretion)
- excessive cardiovascular abnormalities: impaired cardiac function, a decrease of HDL cholesterol, and an increase of LDL cholesterol

Treatment and Dosages

GH is available only by prescription and can be administered only by injection. Patients self-administer the drug before they go to sleep (the best time to release GH in the body). Along with fellow members of the Growth Hormone Research Society, I have found that there is no set formula regarding dose. The rule of thumb is to start with a low dose and gradually increase to the point where IGF-1 concentrations reflect an adequate GH response. I usually start my patients with a 0.4 to 0.5 IU (international unit) as a daily dose. To be effective, GH therapy needs to be given for six months or longer.

Potential Side Effects and Precautions

The older the patient, the more likely he or she will feel some joint pains or stiffness with GH therapy. But the dose usually can be adjusted to eliminate the symptom. Carpal tunnel syndrome (swelling at the underside of the wrist causing pressure on the median nerve with pain, tingling, and numbness of the thumb and index and middle fingers) is very rare if the doses are kept low. Hypertension and blood glucose levels have to be checked. Gynecomastia (the growth of breast tissue in men) has been reported in scientific literature as a possible side effect, although in my four years of experience with GH therapy, I have never seen it. Cancer is a concern if the patient has had a recent tumor, but the risk of cancer is not increased.

In general, the bad press GH has received has been because of researchers who used massive doses. However, patients with the following conditions should avoid GH therapy: active cancer, chronic edema, active carpal tunnel syndrome, uncontrolled hypertension, pregnancy, a fasting blood glucose level of more than 120–130, and diabetes.

Natural Growth Hormone Releasers

Most older people have enough GH in storage in the pituitary gland; it just needs to be released. Previously, amino acids such as arginine and lysine were promoted as having the ability to induce GH release. In my clinical experience, L-glutamine offers the best approach. There's no guarantee that even L-glutamine will release GH, but should it fail to do so, you would still receive additional benefits. L-glutamine can help repair the lining of the intestinal tract, enhance the production of internal natural antioxidant glutathione, and build muscle tissue. Begin by taking 2 grams daily at bedtime. If there are no side effects, such as nausea, diarrhea, or upset stomach, then increase up to 5 grams. To quantify the results, have your physician measure your IGF-1 levels before and then after one or two weeks of the program.

Things to Avoid

There is an inverse relationship between high blood sugar levels and the release of growth hormone; therefore you should:

- ◆ avoid sugary foods. There is no better way to elevate your blood sugar levels than by consuming a bag of jelly beans or a big piece of cake slathered with frosting. The worst culprits are foods that have a very high ratio of sugar to fiber.
- ◆ avoid sweet snacks before bedtime. GH is released mainly while you sleep. Eating something sweet (even a little sweet) results in an elevated blood sugar level that can last for hours, even in a person with a normal glucose metabolism.
- ◆ avoid eating before exercising. Exercise induces a release of GH. Eating right before working out elevates blood sugar and may negate the effect.

On the Horizon: Growth Hormone Pills and Patches

If the prospect of daily injections of GH leaves you cold, you'll be happy to hear that several new kinds of GH-releasing agents are being tested which will be administered by a pill or a transdermal skin patch. They should be on the market by the year 2000.

When these new GH-releasing agents were discovered, a new brain endocrine physiology—a new cell receptor—was discovered along with them. The scientific world is anxiously waiting to see who will be the first to discover the never previously identified hormone that fits into this receptor. How does this still-to-be discovered hormone interact with GH? Perhaps a Nobel Prize will go to the discoverer.

6

The Four Dimensions of Aging

When I first met Jackie Joyner-Kersee, she was an eighteen-year-old freshman who had come to UCLA to play basketball. After establishing that she could do that exceedingly well, she decided to test her talents in track and field. In an amazingly short time she was competing in the most difficult endeavor, the heptathlon, comprised of seven different events: sprinting, distance running, shotput, javelin, high jump, hurdles, and long jump. In the 1984 Olympic Games she took the silver medal in pentathlon, barely missing the gold by a few points. In the 1988 and 1992 Olympic Games, she took home the gold. Her domination in this event, with multiple world records over such a long period, has never been equaled.

With her record of achievements you would never know that Jackie has an illness that can be devastating to an athlete: asthma. By the time I met Jackie, I had already begun to formulate a theory about aging after a long and intensive study. I had concluded that all the various processes of aging in the human body could be explained by changes that occur in three broad categories. Working with Jackie caused me to rethink the theory and add a fourth category. We therefore have these four categories:

1. Neuroendocrine: how hormones and the nervous system signals interrelate
2. Energy Metabolism: how we gain and utilize energy, or the effectiveness of our energy metabolism system
3. Biomechanical: how we move
4. Lifestyle and Environment: the social and personal dynamics that govern our personality and style, and how we relate to one another, the world, and the environment.

Another person with an illness like Jackie's might have dismissed the idea of becoming a competitive athlete. Make no mistake, there were a number of times when her asthma was so severe that it required emergency treatment. But Jackie adapted to her environment and *chose* to succeed despite the pain and adversity.

There is actually another dimension of aging—genes. Your biological parents affect the way you age. But there is little you can do about this dimension of aging, so there is really no practical reason to discuss it. In the next ten to twenty years this fifth dimension of aging will become increasingly important. The Human Genome Project, the international scientific effort to map all 100,000 human genes, is ahead of schedule and has already yielded new therapies for a wide range of diseases associated with aging and others—from breast, prostate, and lung cancer to inserting longevity genes or repairing injured genes to give you an extra thirty or more years of good living beyond your normal life expectancy. Soon many of the diseases and afflictions associated with our advanced years—for example, Alzheimer's and osteoporosis—might be cured by fixing a cell's suboptimal genetic structure. In the meantime, our best strategy is to halt and even reverse the effect of aging by taking full advantage of the antiaging breakthroughs that are imminent. (See chapter 18 for more about future antiaging therapies.)

All of us are dealt a genetic hand with certain physiological advantages and disadvantages. Even with the best training, you may never be capable of winning an Olympic heptathlon or decathlon. But you are capable of reaching your maximum vitality with an integrated anabolic program that addresses the four dimensions of aging.

Each of us is a synergistic biological entity composed of interrelated systems. All these systems age in a different way and for different reasons. And they all affect one another and overlap in un-expected ways. While addressing each is vital for an effective anti-aging program, the four major causes of aging are listed in order of their relative importance.

Dimension of Aging #1: Neuroendocrine

There are two parts of the neuroendocrine system. The "endocrine" part refers to the hormones (discussed in detail in the last chapter). The "neuro" part refers to "neurotransmitters," a term coined in 1904 to describe chemical compounds stored in nerve cells of the brain and other organs. When stimulated, these chemicals cross the gaps between nerve fibers, transmitting messages within the brain and to other parts of the body.

Neurotransmitters and hormones are closely linked: the former controls the release of the latter. Too much or too little of a neuro-transmitter can throw the delicate balance between the hormones into disarray.

As we age, we produce less of many hormones, including the sex hormones, DHEA, growth hormone, thyroid hormone, mela-tonin, as well as neurotransmitters, including dopamine, acetyl-choline, and norepinephrine. Compounding the problem is the decline—both in number and sensitivity—of the receptors in cells that receive the hormones. Even if you have enough of a hormone, the target cells become insensitive to hormone stimulation.

This relationship between neurotransmitters, hormones, and cell receptors is responsible for human behavior, from emotional moods (such as anger or pleasure) to physical feelings (hunger or pain), and movement (arms and legs), involuntary processes (diges-tion, breathing), and cognitive abilities (intellectual understanding, memory).

Neurotransmitters

There have been more than one hundred neurotransmitters identi-fied, but many of them fall into three broad categories: acetyl-choline, dopamine, and serotonin.

ACETYLCHOLINE: Acetylcholine is distributed throughout the body, but in the brain it is involved in the human mind, the mental functions that differentiate us from other mammals. These functions include insight, critical judgment (also called executive function), memory, language, spatial relationships, sensory impressions and interpretations, speech, and thought. Aging leads to declines of the enzyme called choline acetyl-transferase that controls the biosynthesis of acetylcholine from choline and acetyl-coenzyme A.

Full-blown depletion of acetylcholine results in Alzheimer's disease. Alzheimer's is not a normal consequence of aging. Some of us will have some degree of impairment of memory, language, thought, orientation, and critical thinking if we live long enough. This is, however, distinct from Alzheimer's, a very specific disease process seen in older people but *not* a condition present *just* because you are older or aging.

While Alzheimer's is thought to have a significant genetic mechanism associated with it, a number of risk factors increase your likelihood of getting it. They range from trauma to the head (also called boxer's dementia) to couch potato syndrome. Regarding the latter, there is a statistical correlation between a higher level of education and/or a lifetime of ongoing adult intellectual stimulation and the *decreased* risk of Alzheimer's. (More on that in chapter 13.)

DOPAMINE: This category includes, in addition to dopamine, norepinephrine, and epinephrine, which are related to energy release and consumption. These keep us vigilant and alert, controlling the release of adrenaline for the "fight or flight" mechanism that automatically arouses us in an emergency. When stimulated, dopamine makes your heart beat faster, increases your rate of breathing, and generally makes you ready to do battle, flee for your life, or make passionate love. It is also responsible for involuntary movements (such as blinking), emotional drive, and spontaneity.

Dopamine declines with age, but you can also burn it out earlier by taking cocaine, crack, speed, or other stimulants. The "high" from these "uppers" comes from the quick acceleration of dopamine, which is typically followed by an emotional letdown as the body's supply of dopamine is depleted.

Norepinephrine, was at the heart of the revolution in biochemical treatment of depression. Depressed patients, it was discovered, have low levels of norepinephrine, and many antidepressant medications increase the concentration of norepinephrine in the brain.

The majority of the 10 million or so dopamine and related cells are located deep in the brain. As dopamine is used, a very toxic free radical is produced that contributes to the demise of its parent cell, the dopamine neuron. With aging, this activity increases to the point where there are not enough dopamine neurons left to do their important function since new ones aren't being generated. Research on stimulating the growth of new dopamine cells and the creation of additional dopamine is currently in progress.

Dopamine's self-destructive nature can be accelerated by certain medications (such as L-dopa), environmental toxins (exposure to heavy metals), or even lifestyle choices (a pro-oxidative diet and drug abuse). Full-blown dopamine deficiency is known as Parkinson's disease. You have to lose about 75 percent of your dopamine neurons before you have a case of obvious Parkinson's.

A dramatic story about lifestyle-induced destruction of the dopamine neurons concerns a chemical compound called MPTP and a mystery involving two graduate students living on opposite ends of the country: Santa Cruz, California, and Stony Brook, New York. Both students had a nasty little habit—heroin—that they didn't mind sharing with friends for the right price. Coincidentally, they both made the same mistake at about the same time while synthesizing the drug in their illicit labs. They inadvertently created MPTP (1-methyl-4-phenyl-1,2,3,6-tetralydropyridine), which turned out to be extremely toxic to the dopamine neurons. Weeks after using these heroin batches, young addicts were coming to medical facilities on both coasts and presenting the symptoms of classic Parkinson's disease, normally seen in the elderly.

Some scientists are predicting a new wave of Parkinson's as the result of people using cocaine, crack, and other stimulants combined with other pro-oxidants such as smoking, drinking, antioxidant-poor diets, and poor sleep patterns. In this scenario all these factors combine to destroy the dopamine neurons, pushing them into an auto-destruct point of no return. The old wave of Parkinson's disease sufferers, who are now dying off, is thought to have been the result of exposure to industrial chemicals (before today's worker safety and pollution control regulations were instituted) and from a viral encephalitis epidemic that struck millions in the U.S.A. in the 1920s.

SEROTONIN: Serotonin influences appetite, cravings, and obsessive behaviors. A person with low serotonin can be impulsive, aggressive, violent, anxious, restless, and depressed (even suicidal), and exhibits compulsive habits including overeating and drug and alcohol abuse. Too much serotonin can lead to impaired sexual function, including an inability to have an orgasm or an ejaculation, as well as nausea and diarrhea. These are the same side effects associated with the popular drugs Prozac, Paxil, Zoloft, and the others known as SSRIs (Selective Serotonin Reuptake Inhibitors). These drugs block (inhibit) the nerve cell from reabsorbing serotonin once it is released, prolonging the action of the serotonin. Stressed-out people take SSRIs because serotonin, known as the civilizing neurotransmitter, promotes tranquillity and decreases mental activity.

Pregnancy is an excellent example of serotonin dominating the other neurotransmitters. The "glow" that pregnant women exhibit is largely due to their increased levels of serotonin. This is a time when serotonin overrides the effects of norepinephrine, which is excitatory. To preserve the fetus, women sleep more, gain weight, and lower their rate of mental activity. Because of lowered mental activity, there is less pain perception and an increased pain threshold, vital, as your mother can tell you, during birth.

Melatonin is made from serotonin in a two-step process in the pineal gland of the brain. The pineal gland, also called the "seat of the soul" by the ancient Greeks, primarily functions to produce melatonin, which operates as your body's "biological clock." Melatonin production and release is governed mainly by cycles of light and dark (night and day and seasonal)—turned off by daylight and turned on by darkness. The pineal gland and melatonin also regulate the daily rhythmic action of the hypothalamus-pituitary gland cyclical activities. This regulation is the reason for night and day differences and fluctuations in the secretion of growth hormone, testosterone, cortisol, and other hormones.

Serotonin is made in our brain cells during the day as we eat carbohydrates, then gets rapidly converted to melatonin starting at sundown. Melatonin's peak level release is at about 3:00 A.M. Since melatonin affects the main endocrine center of the brain (hypothal-amus-pituitary), it influences a wide range of functions from im-munity to fertility, growth, and insulin production. We don't feel the effects of a low level of melatonin as directly as those of sero-tonin. The effects are subtle and spread out over the twenty-four hours of a day. A big shot of serotonin affects you immediately. A large enough dose of melatonin can do the same, but that is not the way our bodies normally function.

Unlike the other two major neurotransmitter groups, serotonin does not decline dramatically over time (although melatonin secre-tion decreases sharply with age). But because the others do, this creates a greater dominance of serotonin over melatonin, acetyl-choline, and catecholamines. Some scientists theorize this imbal-ance may be a major cause of aging. If you are less than sixty years old and have a serotonin-melatonin imbalance, you will exhibit signs of accelerated aging, including increased stress and cortisol levels, resulting in depression, anxiety, poor sleep, impaired glucose metabolism, and sexual dysfunctions; and/or poor impulse control, leading to behaviors such as drinking, overeating, recklessness, ag-gressiveness, and violent tendencies.

Dimension of Aging #2: Energy Metabolism

There are two components to the energy metabolism system. The first is the delivery of fuel inside the cell, that is, the process of get-ting food from your mouth into the cell. The second is getting fuel into the mitochondria, the cells' power plants which produce the high-energy compounds that cells and muscles need to function.

You derive the maximum and most efficient energy from glu-cose-based fuel sources. If exercise is prolonged and strenuous, then fat products called fatty acids and amino acids are burned (ox-idized) for fuel instead of glucose. An efficiently working metabolic system obtains energy first from glucose/glycogen, and when it has exhausted that fuel, then from fats and proteins.

With age, both of these metabolic functions begin to fall apart. It becomes increasingly difficult to move glucose into the cell, and the mitochondria begin to wear down and work less efficiently.

A primary culprit in this aging process is insulin. A vital anabolic hormone, in excess it becomes dangerous. Normally, insulin serves as the equivalent of a freight train, transporting glucose to the cell. For a number of reasons, however, cells become resistant to insulin with age, essentially preventing it from doing its job. Cut off from its regular fuel supply of glucose, cells have no other choice but to start burning the furniture to keep the furnaces running, that is, the fatty acids from fat stores.

Sounds great, doesn't it? As we get older, we burn less glucose and more fat. What could be wrong with that? Well, back at the train station, the insulin workers are getting itchy. Blocked from doing their glucose-transporting job, the insulin agents begin storing everything you eat as fat. Even though your cells are burning fat instead of glucose, insulin is working even harder to store it, and the net result is that your body fat increases.

The second bit of bad news about insulin is that with age it fails to give the proper signals for the synthesis of proteins (the muscle's building blocks). As a result, you lose muscle mass, which of course worsens the first problem of increasing body fat. If you think this sounds like a formula for middle-age flab, you're right.

The third piece of bad news about insulin is that with age the bloodstream is flooded with excess insulin and glucose. Instead of working together in a productive relationship, insulin and glucose now shun each other and linger in the blood, causing trouble for blood vessels and vital organs such as the eyes, nerves, and kidneys. (The worst-case scenario of the glucose-insulin system breakdown occurs in a condition known as Metabolic Syndrome X and further down the road, diabetes. See page 155 for more information.)

Excess insulin isn't entirely responsible for the energy-metabolism problems that occur with aging. The mitochondria wear down and begin leaking the equivalent of smoke fumes. Imagine two power plants that produce electrical energy from burning gasoline. One is an efficient engine that burns the fuel cleanly with little smoke. The other engine burns the gasoline but produces a lot of smoke and soot, polluting itself and the neighboring area. The already damaged engine damages itself more as it converts one energy source to another. This is what happens with aging and oxidative damage to the mitochondria. The "smoke fumes" in this case are called free radicals, which are the basis for a leading theory of why we age.

Many neurodegenerative diseases such as Alzheimer's, Parkinson's, diabetes, and stress-induced memory damage are the result of the body's energy system failing either at the cell insulin-glucose transport level or at the intracellular level involving the mitochondrial power plants.

Dimension of Aging #3: Biomechanical

This is the system of pumps (heart), pipes (blood vessels), levers (joints), pistons and springs (muscles and tendons), and framing (skeleton, bones). Built for motion, this system deteriorates when not used. A good example of this would be if you stayed in bed for a week. Upon arising, you would experience a quick dose of aging symptoms: stiff joints, weak muscles, shortness of breath, and, if you were tested, a loss of bone mass. Interestingly, astronauts in space experience the same symptoms because of the lack of gravity.

Underutilizing your biomechanical system can have devastating direct and indirect consequences. An intrinsic problem is the stagnation or pooling of body fluids. When fluids are not circulated, they get dirty, like a pond that has no runoff versus a fast-running stream. The stagnation of body fluids makes it easier for bacteria or other invaders such as viruses to camp out in our bodies. Inactivity can also lead to curvature of the spine, brittle bones, creaky joints, and weak muscles, which can increase the risk of falls and injuries.

Dimension of Aging #4: Our Lifestyle Choices

Lifestyle choices play an enormous role in our quality of life as we age. We didn't have a choice of who our parents were. We were not given a choice about the culture we were born into, its values, beliefs, and expectations. The genes and the culture we acquire have a powerful impact on our health, aging, and longevity. In the United States, for example, persons of lower economic status and education have shorter life spans. People whose religion forbids alcohol, caffeine, and smoking (Mormons and Seventh-Day Adventists, for example) have a greater chance for a longer life.

But longevity per se is not the goal of this book. It is not how long you live that ultimately counts but how well you live. Habits, social contacts, family and loved ones, even one's outlook on life play a scientifically verifiable role in the health of everyone, especially as we age. Exercise, diet, and appropriate supplements can modify the genetic hand we were dealt. I will show you how, beginning with the next chapter.

Part II

The Three
Pathways of Aging

ᔐ 7 ᔑ

Your Mind-Body-Spirit Quotient

Our bodies are governed by a complex network of neuro-transmitters and hormones. The way they interrelate—the body's metabolism for energy, its biomechanical system for movement, and, indeed, even how we conduct our lives, our lifestyles—is unique to every individual.

In treating baby boomer–aged patients in my private practice in Santa Monica, California, an unexpected medical pattern emerged. The rate and degree to which my patients lost certain hormones and neurotransmitters created an observable difference in their mental, physical, and emotional well-being. As mentioned earlier, there are parallels between these middle-aged patients and a wide variety of elite athletes with whom I worked at UCLA and during five Olympic Games.

In the case of the elite athletes, a diminished supply of one neu-rotransmitter, which was often caused by overtraining, would throw the other neurotransmitters out of balance. But in the case of my middle-aged patients, the imbalance was not produced by a self-imposed external factor—that is, overtraining—but simply by living, or, to be more precise, how their bodies aged. And that is when I came upon something quite surprising. The symptoms of my middle-aged patients correlated with dysfunctions in neuro-transmitters. For instance, patients who came to me complaining of unexplainable memory loss were low in acetylcholine or had a block in the neurotransmitter pathway. Patients who had a low sex drive and craved stimulants such as speed or cocaine invariably suffered from decreasing levels of dopamine. The patients who complained of restlessness, agitation, or out-of-control impulses were lacking the brain signal serotonin.

Collecting and analyzing the data, I realized that almost everyone fell into one of these three basic categories. Why three? As discussed in chapter 6, the brain governs the body through a complex network of more than one hundred neurotransmitter systems. But science has identified three that have a dominant role: acetylcholine, dopamine, and serotonin. These are often described in biology as the three "classical" neurotransmitters. Because of their importance for the brain's function (and the development by pharmaceutical companies of lucrative prescription drugs that influence them), they have also gotten the lion's share of basic research. Consequently, we know more about them than the other neurotransmitters.

The Three Pathways

Aging tends to follow three pathways that mirror the three classical neurotransmitter systems: a loss of mental (acetylcholine), physical (dopamine), and emotional (serotonin) balance. I refer to these three pathways as Mind, Body, and Spirit.

The Mind Pathway addresses the higher centers of the brain, the executive functions that include cognition, language, memory, and decision-making. The neurotransmitter most closely associated with these functions in the brain is acetylcholine.

The Body Pathway concerns the functional or primitive parts of the brain that control movement, sex drive, physical pleasure, alertness, physical spontaneity, erect posture, reaction time, and overall energy. The system that regulates these basic functions of the body uses the dopamine neurotransmitter.

The Spirit Pathway refers to the system of the brain that regulates mood, appetite, capacity to be civilized, sleeping, sexual behavior, and drug-induced hallucinations. Serotonin is converted to melatonin in the pineal gland. When the serotonin neurotransmitter is working, you feel comfortable, in control, at peace, and you have a restorative sleep pattern. You have a sense of calm and no unusual perplexing needs or desires.

The interrelationships among these neurotransmitters make their functions overlap somewhat. Low serotonin leads to sleeplessness, which leads to low physical energy. Dropping dopamine levels reduces the brain's arousal mechanism, which will eventually affect muscle tone. And with age we lose some of all these neurotransmitters. But it is not the general decline of the neurotransmitter levels nor the loss of their functionality that has the most profound effect on our aging but, rather, the pronounced imbalance of the whole system.

Think of a symphony orchestra in which one section is off-key. If the quality of musicianship overall were to diminish by, say, 10 percent over the course of a season, chances are that only the most discerning critic would notice the difference. But if, beginning with the second performance, the brass section was noticeably off-key, it

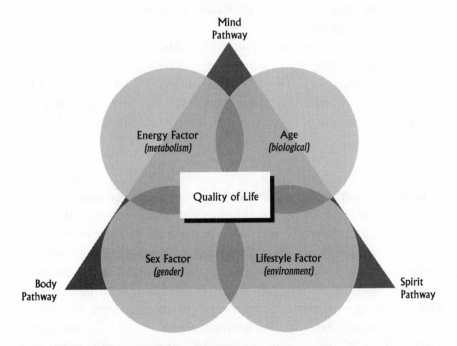

Figure I—"Aging and the Quality of Life"
An integrated antiaging program promotes quality of life by addressing the genetically determined pathways of the brain (Mind, Body, and Spirit) as well as the four primary factors affecting aging: energy metabolism, sex, biological age, and lifestyle.

would immediately impact the performance of the entire orchestra—and everybody would notice the difference. The same is true with our neurotransmitters. One entire section off-key can throw the entire body out of harmony.

On the Way to Building a Personal Antiaging Regimen

In a few moments, you will complete the first of a series of questionnaires designed to help you build your own individual Personal Antiaging Regimen. The first one, the Mind-Body-Spirit Quotient, will determine which of the three pathways you belong on. After completing the Mind-Body-Spirit Quotient questionnaire, you will be directed to chapter 8, 9, or 10 for antiaging advice that is specific to your particular pathway. The advice covers nutritional supplements, diet, exercise, and prescription medications as well as lifestyle recommendations.

In subsequent chapters you will further customize your Personal Antiaging Regimen by answering questions that relate to energy metabolism, sex, lifestyle, and biological age. At the end of this process you will have a very good idea of how to reduce and decrease the effects of aging for your individual physiology.

Cautions

Let me emphasize here that the best way to utilize your Personal Antiaging Regimen is in consultation with a knowledgeable health care professional. While this book is the first to look at the aging process as it affects the individual and his or her unique pathway of aging, nothing replaces a diagnosis by an informed health care professional. Before embarking on *any* major change in diet or exercise, or using nutritional supplements or medications, you should first have a complete medical history, physical and laboratory evaluation. If you are taking medication, consult a physician as to whether a recommended supplement might conflict in any way. Throughout the text, supplements that might be particularly problematic for certain preexisting conditions have been red-flagged.

An important note about supplements: The supplements recommended in chapters 8, 9, and 10 are based on a model of what is needed by an average forty-five-year-old man or woman of normal body proportions to increase his or her anabolic (antiaging) drive. This is only the first step in creating your Personal Antiaging Regimen. It is important to finish the formula by factoring in your Energy Factor (chapter 11), Sex Factor (chapter 12), Lifestyle Factor (chapter 13), and Age Factor (chapter 14).

Because each of us has a unique physiology, it's impossible to determine the exact dosage or program appropriate for everyone. Always follow this rule when taking supplements: *Start low and go slow.* If you find the dosages of the supplements are not effective, *gradually* adjust them higher. It is important to remember that when taking supplements that affect your mental performance and when adding a new smart mood-affecting supplement, it can reduce the need for other smart nutrients. Often these agents act in harmony or synergy, and the additive effects can be more than what you need.

The smart, or *nootropic,* agents, which are sometimes dramatic in effect, have to be adjusted more slowly. The smart agents also tend to work at different speeds. For instance, ginkgo biloba takes one to three months for most people to feel its effect. Give these supplements a three-month trial before abandoning them.

The amount or degree of increase in doses is determined by the agent and the effect needed. There is no set dosage that works for each substance. The amount of increase is dictated by the incremental units available. Sometimes it is 5- to 25-milligram (mg) increments or 50–100 micrograms (mcg) or 50–100 international units (IU). It is always safest to increase with the smallest possible unit of change available.

Some people have such a high degree of hormonal/neurotransmitter disharmony that drastic measures need to be taken. A corrective phase can be employed to jump-start the entry phase of treatment to produce an immediate effect. Later, the corrective phase is scaled back to a maintenance phase that will still produce a long-term antiaging effect. This type of intensive program must be administered by a qualified health care professional.

Fighting the Four "Downers"

No matter which aging pathway you find yourself on, there are supplements that everybody over thirty-five should take as part of their antiaging regimen. Consider this the foundation on which to construct your customized house that will protect you from the ravages of aging. These supplements have been shown to retard various aspects of aging and represent in real terms the tangible results of the tremendous progress made in antiaging research in the last two decades. Will taking supplements allow you to live forever? No. But they will help fight the four "downers" of aging—discomfort, drugs, disability, and doctors—that most people experience in the last phases of their lives.

What is the disadvantage of taking these supplements? There is none. None of these supplements, taken in the prescribed amounts, are toxic in any way. The cost will vary depending on where you buy them, whether you want the very best possible formulation (those that have the best solubility, absorption, and bioavailability) or the average, and what you can afford to invest. Personally, I can't imagine how money could be better spent.

The list of supplements in our "Antiaging Cocktail" might seem daunting at first glance, but keep in mind that many of these recommended nutrients are packaged together in various combinations. Many popular brand-name supplements, such as Centrum, One-A-Day, and Forward, contain twenty-five or more ingredients.

To replicate the Antiaging Cocktail you'll have to do a little homework. Compare one brand against the next until you have a combination of supplements containing all the nutrients in their recommended dosages. It may be difficult to match the recommended doses exactly, so do the best you can. For convenience, the Antiaging Cocktail is broken down into broad categories according to their functions. Antioxidants, for example, which fight the catabolic (pro-aging) free radicals, are an essential element in your regimen. The mitochondrial protectors, the so-called B vitamins, "smart oils," and herbs and spices, play important roles as well. If you want to know more about the function of each individual supplement in the Antiaging Cocktail, turn to chapter 16.

The recommended dosages for the supplements in the Antiaging Cocktail are the basic amounts required to be effective for the problems and programs presented in this book. Some of the ingredients can be modified upward for various reasons: increased physical activity (you're training for a marathon), decreased nutritional status (your work demands that you skip lunch), or increased pollution (exposure to toxins, smoking, alcohol abuse) and others. Follow the instructions in your pathway regimen for possible increased dosages. These supplements are to be taken once a day, any time of day, with or without food, unless otherwise noted. In addition to antiaging nutrients, the formula includes essential general health nutrients not known to have specific antiaging effects.

Diet and Exercise as Part of Your Regimen

Supplements are an essential part of your antiaging regimen, which numerous research studies have shown and my own two decades of clinical experience confirm, but there are still health care professionals who believe that a well-balanced diet is all you need to maintain proper health, no matter what your age. Even qualified nutritional scientists will disagree as to what constitutes a "well-balanced diet." Also, there is a great deal of individual genetic variation that influences how we absorb, tolerate, and utilize different foods.

You and I belong to another school of thought. We believe in taking advantage of every opportunity to maintain our health and vigor.

A proper nutrient-rich diet and an appropriate exercise program are vital components of your antiaging regimen. Both are important mechanisms for releasing the growth hormone. Yes, you would still be ahead of the aging game if you did nothing but follow the recommendation for supplements in this book. But our goal is to take advantage of every avenue that will keep you youthful until antiaging science and technology soon after the turn of the century reward us with new and astonishing methods for slowing the aging process.

Why are exercise and diet so important? Let's take them one at a time. In chapter 6 we discussed how the key to your aging profile is found in the body's four dimensions of aging. Among these is the biomechanical dimension—the joints, bones, and muscles, which allow us to move. When this system suffers, it throws off the entire body. An unfit biomechanical system will lead to decreased mobility, resulting in loss of joint mobility, lung capacity, cardiovascular health, and tissue contraction, which in turn lead to a stagnation effect on the circulation of body fluids (blood, lymph, spinal fluid). Think of a sedentary life as what happens when water in a pond is allowed to stagnate. The ecosystem dies. Now compare that to a quickly running stream with its rich and healthy ecology.

Diet is a little more complicated. You may not exercise no matter how many times you're told it's good for you, but we both know you will eat. How you eat and what and when can have a dramatic impact on your aging process in two ways. By eating "dumb" you can increase the catabolic direction of the body to produce excessive amounts of insulin and free radicals. This is especially true for those with a genetic inclination toward an abnormal energy metabolism. (You will find out more about this when you take your Energy Factor in chapter 11.) By eating "smart" you can decrease the catabolic processes by supplying your body with nutrients to help rebalance the neurological messengers—the neurotransmitters—returning them to their youthful ratios.

Supplements to a large degree can provide these nutrients, but some nutrients are best obtained through diet—lycopene, for example, a potent antioxidant found in tomatoes. There are lycopene supplements available, but when a food nutrient is extracted from its host, we miss the synergistic effect of the whole food.

There's not one "right" diet for everybody. The diet best for you depends on both your aging profile (your Mind-Body-Spirit Quotient) and your glucose-metabolism profile (your Energy Factor). You've noticed how the claims of various diet books on the market conflict. One will recommend a high-protein diet, another a high-carbohydrate diet. (We're still waiting for *The All-Fat Diet Book,* which no doubt would be an instant best-seller!) In a sense, they're all right. For some individuals, a high-protein diet is right; for others, a high-carb diet; and, yes, for some a diet with a relatively high-fat ratio. The key to maximizing your diet and exercise is to follow the program that is right for you.

THE MIND-BODY-SPIRIT QUOTIENT

The following three-part questionnaire is designed to determine your primary pathway of aging: Mind (deficiency in acetylcholine), Body (deficiency in dopamine, or Spirit (deficiency in serotonin). Answer *every* question yes or no to the best of your ability. If the answer to a question is yes, write the corresponding points in the blank at the beginning of each question. Score 0 if the answer is no.

Mind Pathway

___ 1. Does your family have a history of Alzheimer's disease occurring before age 65? If yes, score 4 points.

___ 2. . . . after age 65? If yes, score 3 points.

___ 3. Have you ever had multiple head injuries? If yes, score 2 points.

___ 4. Have you ever had an inflammation of the brain, such as encephalitis, or other inflammatory condition of the brain or nervous system? If yes, score 2 points.

___ 5. Do you regularly use aluminum cookware or aluminum-containing antacids such as Alternagel? If yes, score 2 points.

___ 6. Are you someone who has ongoing food allergies or allergies in general? If yes, score 2 points.

___ 7. Have you ever been significantly exposed to heavy metals, such as lead, mercury, cadmium, and so forth? If yes, score 3 points.

___ 8. Have you ever been told you have high blood levels of a substance called homocysteine? If yes, score 3 points.

___ 9. Are you a woman who has decided not to take estrogen replacement therapy despite loss of your ovarian function from menopause, surgery, or another cause? If yes, score 3 points.

___ 10. If your sex is female, score 2 points.

___ 11. Are you experiencing problems with recent memory retention? Do you repeatedly forget what you did or what you were going to do in the past 30 minutes to 1 hour? If yes, score 2 points.

___ 12. Did you have difficulty obtaining a high school diploma? If yes, score 1 point.

___ 13. Have you noticed that it is increasingly difficult to follow a plot in a television show or a movie? If yes, score 2 points.

___ 14. Is it becoming harder for you to do things that require mathematical skills, such as paying the bills or balancing the checkbook? If yes, score 2 points.

___ 15. Have persons close to you mentioned that you don't seem to be yourself or that your personality has changed? If yes, score 1 point.

___ 16. You will need a clock or a watch plus a pen to take the following 1-minute test: Name 12 items that begin with the letter "D."

1. _____

2. _____

3. _____

4. _____

5. _____

6. _____

7. _____

8. _____

9. _____

10. _____

11. _____

12. _____

Score 1 point if you wrote less than 12. Score 2 points if you wrote less than 6.

___ 17. Have you noticed that it is increasingly difficult to understand or remember something you have just read? If yes, score 2 points.

___ 18. Do you sometimes not know where you are going or get lost? If yes, score 2 points.

___ 19. Is it getting harder to learn new things? If yes, score 2 points.

___ 20. Have your friends commented that you seem to be more moody, more irritable, or less concerned? If yes, score 1 point.

___ 21. Do you find yourself unable to make up your mind or reach a decision about simple matters? If yes, score 1 point.

___ 22. Has there been a slow decline in your ability to form new ideas and think creatively? If yes, score 2 points.

___ 23. Have you been told that your memory is getting worse? If yes, score 2 points.

Add up your score and write it below:
MIND—Total Score: ____

Body Pathway

___ 1. Do you have a family history of Parkinson's disease? If yes, score 4 points.

___ 2. If you are male, score 3 points.

___ 3. Are you experiencing an overall slowing of movement? If yes, score 2 points.

___ 4. Look in a mirror and study your face for a moment. Does it appear that even when you try, your face lacks emotion, expressiveness? Is it vacant looking? If yes, score 2 points.

___ 5. Do you *feel* tired and listless most or all of the time? If yes, score 1 point.

___ 6. Do you find it increasingly difficult to initiate new projects? If yes, score 2 points.

___ 7. Is it difficult for you to respond emotionally to situations or events? If yes, score 1 point.

___ 8. Do you find yourself losing balance, stumbling, and bumping into things more than ever? If yes, score 2 points.

___ 9. Take these quick dexterity tests:
(a) Tap your thumb against your index finger 10 times as widely and as fast as possible.
(b) Open your hand as wide as possible and close it as fast as possible 10 times.

Did you find it difficult to maintain a wide range of motion or arc of motion and a constant rapid speed? Score 3 points for each test that you answer yes.

___ 10. Are you noticing a decreased sex interest or drive? If yes, score 1 point.

___ 11. These questions are about how you walk. If you are not sure of the answers, ask a friend to look at how you walk.

(a) Is your posture stooped forward or does it go off to one side? If yes, score 3 points.

(b) Does your gait have short and shuffling steps? If yes, score 3 points.

(c) Do you swing your arms out widely from the body when striding (walking fast)? If *no*, score 2 points.

___ 12. Do your arms and legs feel rigid or stiff when you move them? If yes, score 2 points.

___ 13. Do you experience involuntary movement, tremors, or shaking of your hands and fingers while not actively using them? If yes, score 3 points.

___ 14. Do you feel as if your muscles are growing weaker? Is it more difficult to pick up or lift objects, crouch down, or get out of bed? If yes, score 1 point.

___ 15. Have you noticed that your reaction time has decreased, for example, when you're driving? If yes, score 1 point.

___ 16. Have you or others noticed your speech tone becoming flatter or monotone? If this is too difficult to answer, ask a friend to assess you. If yes, score 2 points.

___ 17. Do you feel a general lack of emotion toward people, including loved ones and family? If yes, score 1 point.

___ 18. Do you find it increasingly difficult to wake up or stay alert after drinking a cup of coffee that has caffeine? Does it take 2 or 3 cups to stay alert when previously 1 cup did the trick? If yes, score 1 point.

___ 19. Do you take an iron supplement (such as Geritol) or a vitamin with an iron supplement, or have you cooked with iron pots or taken iron injections? If yes, score 2 points.

___ 20. Do you find it difficult to start or initiate movements of your body? If yes, score 3 points.

___ 21. Have you ever been repeatedly exposed to a lot of pesticides? If yes, score 3 points.

Add up your score and write it below:
BODY—Total Score: _____

Spirit Pathway

___ 1. Are you intermittently anxious for no apparent reason? If yes, score 1 point.

___ 2. Do you feel more calm and relaxed after eating pure carbohydrates such as plain bagels, puffed rice crackers, or French bread on an empty stomach? If yes, score 2 points.

___ 3. Do you suffer from seasonal depression, particularly in the fall or winter? If yes, score 3 points.

___ 4. Is your sleep generally characterized by restless nights punctuated by frequent wakings? If yes, score 2 points.

___ 5. Do you feel tired when you wake? If yes, score 1 point.

___ 6. Do you have repeated episodes of high irritability, leading to aggressiveness or losing your temper frequently? If yes, score 3 points.

___ 7. Do you need to take a drug or alcohol to feel better more than just on an occasion? If so, score 3 points.

___ 8. Do you tend to be obsessive or compulsive in your daily habits to a degree that it bothers you or others? If yes, score 3 points.

___ 9. Do you feel apathetic about life? Is it difficult to enjoy activities you used to find fun and rewarding? Are you bothered constantly by negative thoughts such as suicide? If yes, score 3 points.

___ 10. Do you find yourself being more sexual than you care to be? Do you feel burdened by constant, overwhelming, or uncontrolled sexual desires or fantasies? If yes, score 2 points.

___ 11. Do you frequently binge and desire sugary or starchy types of foods (white bread, bagels, rice cakes, sweet rolls, donuts, and so forth? If yes, score 1 point.

___ 12. Do you lose control when gambling and can't stop? If yes, score 3 points.

___ 13. Have you ever been treated for overeating? If yes, score 3 points.

___ 14. Do you have recurrent episodes of aching or pain or tender areas in your muscles, bones, or joints for no apparent reason? If yes, score 2 points.

___ 15. Do you have a recurring problem with falling asleep and staying asleep? If yes, score 2 points.

___ 16. Do you have recurring thoughts or fears that you have some terrible medical condition? If yes, score 3 points.

____ 17. Do you have a recurring problem of being overweight by more than 20 pounds? If yes, score 2 points.

Add up your score and write it below.
SPIRIT—Total Score: _____

INTERPRETING YOUR SCORES

Determining Your Aging Pathway

Compare the total scores for each of the three sections of the Mind-Body-Spirit Quotient. The section with the highest score determines your probable aging pathway. For example, if the highest of your three scores was in Part II, Body, then you are most likely on the Body Pathway, meaning that to some degree you are experiencing a deficiency in the dopamine neurotransmitter system. Those scoring highest on Part I, Mind, are at risk of having a deficiency in the acetylcholine neurotransmitter signals. And those scoring highest on Part III: Spirit Pathway, have a tendency toward a dysfunction in the serotonin neurotransmitter system.

Determining your Pathway is the first step in customizing your Personal Antiaging Regimen. To learn more about your pathway type, turn to chapter 8 for Mind Pathway; chapter 9 for Body Pathway; or chapter 10 for Spirit Pathway.

Determining Your Degree of Mind-Body-Spirit Aging

Combine all three pathway scores and divide by 3. This quotient along with your Age Factor (chapter 14) are indicators of how currently you are aging overall. Use this score as a benchmark to track your progress after you have begun your Personal Antiaging Regimen. If your scores are high in two or more categories, you may be on an advanced aging pathway. Turn first to the chapter about the pathway whose score is the highest, but also review the other relevant chapter(s).

Score

0–35 Low to Normal Aging: Your score indicates that you are not yet experiencing the effects of aging, which means that you were born with great genes, that you've been living an actively healthy lifestyle, or that you're simply not old enough yet for your body to enter into a catabolic or chaotic state. Nevertheless, if you are older than 35, you should consult the chapter about your pathway to see how specifically you can maintain your health as you grow older.

36–75   Mild Aging: You are beginning to experience the effects of aging, in case you haven't noticed. This is a good time to stop taking your body for granted and start actively intervening to keep it vigorous and healthy and slow down the aging processes. Turn to your pathway chapter for specific advice.

76–100   Moderate Aging: You are feeling the results—physically, mentally, and emotionally—of the disease called aging. Twenty years ago your weapons to fight aging were limited pretty much to disease-specific pharmaceuticals, diet, and exercise. Today we have an entire arsenal of anabolic (antiaging) nutrients, along with a much better understanding of how diet and exercise impact the aging process. By creating your Personal Antiaging Regimen, you can actually slow down and even reverse the aging process.

More than 100   *Advanced Aging Track:* You are likely on an accelerated aging path and need immediate intervention. Follow the prescriptive advice in this book and work with a knowledgeable health care professional in building a regimen that may include pharmaceuticals such as growth hormone or other intensive interventions. Consult your pathway chapter for more advice.

The Antiaging Cocktail

Use this list as the foundation for your antiaging supplement regimen. It may look daunting, but don't worry! Most brand-name antioxidant/multivitamin supplements contain many of these ingredients. However, you won't find one supplement that contains all of them. The goal is to try to get a range of supplements that comes closest to this ideal. In subsequent chapters, you will tweak this list here and there as we fine-tune your antiaging program.

Antioxidant Supplements

This group of vitamins, minerals, and phytonutrient antioxidants has been shown in scientific studies to fight one of the leading causes of aging, the production of free radicals, a damaging by-product of metabolism that increases as we age.

- vitamin A (retinol), 5,000 IU
- natural mixed carotenes with beta-carotene, 5–20 mg
- natural vitamin E (with gamma tocopherol), 400–1,000 IU
- vitamin C (Ester C or buffered C), 500–1,000 mg two to three times daily
- flavonoid mixture containing:
  - grape seed extract, 50–300 mg
  - green tea extract (decaffeinated and standardized), 150 mg, one to three times daily
  - mixed bioflavonoid complex with quercetin: 500 mg to 1 gram, twice daily
- minerals/metals supporting the antioxidant enzymes:
  - zinc (chelate), 15–55 mg
  - copper (chelate), 1–3 mg
  - manganese (chelate), 5–15 mg
  - selenium (chelate), 100–500 mcg

Mitochondrial Protectors

Every cell in the human body has tiny power plants called the mitochondria that generate most of the body's energy. Wtih age the mitochondria become damaged for a number of reasons, including exposure to toxic chemicals, leakage of its membranes and attack by its own or other free radicals. The following agents have been shown to protect the mitochondria from effects of degeneration associated with aging.

- CoQ10, 30–300 mg with food or with vitamin E
- acetyl L-carnitine (ALC), 100–2,000 mg before a meal in the daytime
- alpha lipoic acid, 50–600 mg
- N-Acetyl-cysteine, 100–1,200 mg

B Vitamins

The term "B vitamins" describes chemically similar nutrients that are among the most potent antiagers. Their individual functions are described in chapter 16, but among their reported benefits are decreased incidence of heart disease, senility, cancer, depression, and preservation of memory and the immune system. These nutrients are frequently referred to by their individual names, which are indicated by parentheses in the following list:

- B$_1$ (thiamine), 50–100 mg, one to two times daily
- B$_2$ (riboflavin), 10–20 mg, one to two times daily
- B$_3$ (niacinamide), 20–200 mg, one to two times daily
- B$_5$ (pantothenate), 250 mg, one to two times daily
- B$_6$ (pyridoxine), 25–50 mg, one to two times daily
- B$_{12}$ (sublingual methyl cobalamin or coenzymated form), 500 mcg, one to two times daily
- folic acid (always take with B$_{12}$), 400–500 mcg, one to two times daily

Macrominerals

- calcium (chelate), 200–600 mg, twice daily
- magnesium (chelate), 250–800 mg

Trace Minerals

- chromium (nicotinate), 200–400 mcg
- molybdenum (trioxide or sodium molybdate), 50–600 mcg

Miscellaneous

- betaine HCL, 100–150 mg
- vitamin D$_3$, 400–800 IU
- vitamin K$_1$ (phytonadione), 60–300 mcg
- biotin, 100–300 mcg
- inositol, 30–100 mg
- iodine, 50–150 mcg
- boron, 1–6 mg
- potassium, 200–500 mg
- Choline (bitartrate) 250–500 mg

Herbs and Spices

Once dismissed as the products of old wives' tales, herbs and spices are now recognized by researchers for their medicinal phytonutrient properties. What is more, food tastes better with them. Use them liberally, but unless you have an unusually spicy diet, you will probably need to take supplements.

◆ Garlic, one to 2 cloves (4 grams), two to three times daily, or one to two capsules (10 mg allicin or 4,000 mcg total allicin potential), two to three times daily after a meal
◆ season food liberally with cayenne (hot chili peppers), fresh-cracked black pepper, turmeric (curry powder), and fresh parsley
◆ gingko biloba (standardized extract), 40–80 mg, one to three times daily

Smart Oils

◆ high-lignan refrigerated flaxseed oil or EPA-DHA fish oil, one to two tablespoons daily

The Skinny on Smart Oils

Our brains are largely composed of fat. What is more, the cells of the brain utilize fat from our diet. If too much of the wrong kind of fat is eaten, it can induce the lipid-rich parts of the brain to oxidize or break down, similar to the rancidity reaction that occurs when a can of shortening is left on the shelf too long.

Make this one of your antiaging mantras: *Hydrogenated or partially hydrogenated oil equals bad oil.*

Hydrogenated oils or solid vegetable oils do not occur in nature; they're a product of modern industry, which uses them to add taste and texture to a variety of packaged foods, including crackers, cookies, doughnuts, as well as most fried fast food. Hydrogenated oils promote the inflammation and deterioration of brain cells—and this is food for thought the next time you munch a bunch of Mc-Donald's fries.

What is the most common hyrogenated fat? It's probably in your refrigerator now: margarine. But not all fats and oils are bad for you. Monosaturated fats (such as olive oil) are not only slow to oxidize (turn rancid) but actually may fight the effects of free radicals. Unless you get most of your dietary protein from fish, you should take flaxseed oil or fish oil with food and always along with or after your daily vitamin E supplement.

Finding the Right Health Care Professional

Whether he is an M.D., D.O., Ph.D., N.D., chiropractor, dietician, or herbalist, don't necessarily assume your doctor is knowledgeable about or even friendly to the concept of antiaging medicine. How can you tell if your health care professional is an appropriate partner in managing your antiaging regimen? Ask him the following questions. If he answers "no" or "don't know" to most of them, then you have the wrong health partner.

1. Do you know what a smart drug is?
2. What's the difference between a sixties radical and a free radical?
3. Who is Dr. Hayflick, and why is he important?
4. Is it natural to tinker with the human genetic code?
5. Is it morally wrong to make someone young again?
6. Do you feel that people who take DHEA are nuts?
7. Have you heard of the telomere theory of aging?
8. Is there any value in eating soybeans to stay younger?
9. Is it worth the time and effort to take flaxseed oil or garlic capsules?
10. Do I need to take anything except a Centrum or One-A-Day vitamin to keep healthy and fit?

One last clue: If your doctor looks substantially older than his chronological age or is extremely obese, consider changing doctors. Where can you get a reliable recommendation for a qualified health care professional versed in antiaging medicine in your area? Consult Antiaging Physicians in the appendix.

~ 8 ~

Mind Pathway

In many ways the extreme expression of the Mind Pathway aging type is everybody's idea of the elderly. Certainly, Hollywood has depicted this profile of aging over and over again. It's Coach on *Cheers* and Aunt Clara on *Bewitched*. These characters tend to be forgetful and a little scattered in their cognitive abilities but lovable all the same. On a more serious note, the Mind Pathway types can be prime candidates for being on an Alzheimer's-like disease track of mental decline. A severe depletion and dysfunction of the acetylcholine mind-memory system is characteristic of Alzheimer's dementia sufferers.

Based on your Mind-Body-Spirit Quotient score, you appear to be heading down an aging pathway in which your mental faculties might be compromised. Do you notice that you are becoming more forgetful? Is it more difficult to learn new material or to follow an instruction manual? Do you feel that you don't have the ability to make the right decisions about your life? Do you feel increasingly out of touch with the world around you? Visually, are shapes and configurations difficult to differentiate? Do you have problems copying shapes such as triangles and rectangles? Are you as intuitive or insightful as you used to be? Do you have fewer ideas or new thoughts than you once had? Do you have a difficult time concentrating on one project at a time? Do you seem to be frequently at a loss for words? Is it sometimes hard to find names for objects, that is, you know what you want to say but can't get it out? Do persons close to you say you are acting differently? Do you have a problem organizing things, such as paying bills?

These can all be telltale signs of increased disruption, dysfunction, or decline of the acetylcholine system. As we learned in chapter 7, acetylcholine is one of the primary chemical neurotransmitters for maintaining a healthy and efficient memory system. Acetylcholine is essential, in particular, for the brain's cognitive abilities—our memory and our intellect. Acetylcholine metabolism tends to peak at age thirty-five or forty and then begins a gradual decline.

Acetylcholine declines with age in all of us, but in the Mind Pathway types the decline is pronounced and occurs earlier than expected. Rapidly declining acetylcholine neurons result in decreased capacity for memory, thoughts, sensory perception, and the general ability to be involved in events around us.

Mind Pathway types may also experience a decline in libido—or, in some cases, an increased but inappropriate libido. Sex for your partner may seem impersonal and lack intimacy. Physically, there may be nothing wrong with your sexual prowess, but it can be out of control and inappropriate. In instances of depression associated with the Mind Pathway, you may not be interested in having sex anymore.

Your Antiaging Regimen

Supplements

An effective antiaging strategy for the Mind Pathway aging profile must begin with a strong component that supports the brain mitochondrial function. By keeping the cell energy centers (mitochondria) healthy and functioning properly, brain degeneration can be prevented or, at the very least, slowed down.

Among the effective mitochondria protectors is a "smart agent" called acetyl L-carnitine, or ALC. (A smart agent is a nonprescriptive supplement that can promote memory, mood, IQ, perception, and so on.) ALC is normally found in the inner membrane of the mitochondria; its function is to move fats into the mitochondria for energy production. It also serves as a chemical foundation for the primary Mind Pathway neurotransmitter acetylcholine.

As a mitochondria protector, ALC makes the engines in these cellular energy factories work more efficiently and cleaner, producing fewer waste by-products, those dangerous little free radicals. A leading theory of aging suggests that free radicals cause widespread deterioration to the body's mitochondria but especially to the brain's. The most extreme stage of this degeneration is Alzheimer's disease. ALC is thought to prevent this decay if begun early enough, and it has proven to be particularly effective in enhancing memory. Unfortunately, ALC has not proven very effective in improving memory or other problems in the late stage of Alzheimer's.

ALC is included in the all-purpose Antiaging Cocktail. Mind Pathway types should increase the dosage to 1 to 2 grams daily. Take it in the morning before breakfast, since it can have a stimulating effect that might keep you awake if you take it late in the day.

Caution: Women should not take ALC if pregnant or breast-feeding. Other mitochondria-protecting supplements in the Antiaging Cocktail include CoQ10 and alpha lipoic acid. (See chapter 16 for additional information.)

Lecithin is another substance that converts into the primary Mind Pathway neurotransmitter acetylcholine and also has been shown to improve memory. I recommend including it in your supplement regimen. Be sure to take it *with* the B vitamin group in the Antiaging Cocktail since it won't convert to acetylcholine otherwise. Use the new 95 percent phosphatidyl choline form of lecithin.

About 10 percent of men ages forty to sixty and 20 percent of men ages sixty-nine to eighty require testosterone replacement therapy. An inadequate reserve of natural testosterone affects mood, muscles, bones, and cognitive/memory capacity. The male brain needs a reservoir of testosterone to allow the brain to convert it to estrogen for nerve and mind health.

B vitamins have a special relationship to the healthy functioning of the brain. If their supply is deficient enough, you can literally lose your mind—and experience depression, loss of memory, and even dementia. In fact, early senility has been linked to a B vitamin deficiency. One study suggests that 50 percent of all Americans over sixty exhibit some signs of senility due to a lack of some B vitamins. It is believed that B vitamins are so important to brain functioning because they can neutralize a blood protein called *homocysteine,* which in high levels can damage blood vessels and cause damage to the brain and heart. B vitamins are also essential in the formation of all the neurotransmitters.

Another defense is *phosphatidylserine,* a compound of phosphorus and fat in the brain that stimulates the production of acetylcholine and brain cell membrane activity. Memory and learning abilities depend on a continuous supply of this compound, which declines with aging but especially in Mind Pathway types. *Caution:* Consult with a physician if you are taking this substance with anticoagulants because there might be a negative interaction.

We end our discussion of Mind Pathway supplements with DMAE *(dimethylaminoethanol),* a source of choline, one of the B-complex vitamins that is a building block for acetylcholine. We discuss below how certain foods are rich in choline, but it is difficult to get enough choline to replenish a depleted supply. Too much choline-rich food can also cause diarrhea.

DMAE, like ALC, is a smart supplement now available directly to consumers. Studies have shown that as much as 900 milligrams can be taken daily without any harmful side effect, but 300 milligrams twice a day is sufficient for most Mind Pathway types. Consult with a knowledgeable health care professional before taking more. *Caution:* Those with epilepsy or a history of convulsions should not take DMAE.

All the supplements are available over the counter at most health food stores and from mail order supplement and pharmaceutical suppliers. See the Regimen Recap on page 103 for dosage recommendations. See Antiaging Supplement Suppliers in the appendix for items not available at your local drugstore.

Gender Modifier

Solid scientific evidence has emerged that women are more likely than men to be Mind Pathway types. This is especially true for those women who do not replace estrogen, which protects and regenerates neurons, that has been lost because of illness, surgical removal of the ovaries, or menopause. These women can show accentuated memory impairment and other signs and symptoms of accelerated Mind Pathway decline.

For men, an adequate supply of testosterone is needed to

counter the effects of Mind Pathway deficiency because testosterone is a source of estrogen; the conversion of testosterone to estrogen occurs in the brain of both men and women.

For more information on the need for sex hormone replacement therapy, see chapter 12.

Exercise

Mind Pathway types have problems with cognition, language, spatial relations, and recall. They need exercises that coordinate the mind and body, and promote language and recall skills. Examples of these interactive exercises include the martial arts (especially tai chi and kundalini yoga if they involve another person), tennis, badminton, volleyball, and, in fact, most team sports that require a degree of strategizing and coordination with a "game plan." A workout of about one hour, two to three times a week, is recommended. As always, if you're just beginning an exercise program after a long period of being sedentary, begin your physical regimen gradually. If you have any existing health problems, consult with your physician first.

Beyond physical exercise, games involving mental exercise are highly recommended. Chess, Scrabble, bridge, and other games that involve strategizing help sharpen the memory skills.

Diet

Since Mind Pathway types are on an advanced aging track, we want to flood their diet with antiaging phytonutrients and naturally occurring antioxidants, particularly those that enhance cognitive abilities and protect brain cells.

As we learned earlier, the B vitamin group plays a vital role in preserving the mind's cognitive abilities. Foods high in B_1, B_5, B_6, and choline include milk and dairy products, non-white-meat fish (salmon, mackerel, tuna, sardines, trout), eggs (especially yolks), poultry, wheat germ, peanuts, peanut butter, oatmeal, soybeans (including soy burgers, tofu, and soy milk), sweet potatoes, collard greens, lentils, green beans, garbanzo beans, avocado, Brazil nuts, pecans, and sunflower seeds. Overall, the two most effective non-animal-based sources for enhancing memory and other cognitive functions are peanuts and soybeans.

There is evidence that choline—an important substance for Mind Pathway types—breaks down after exercise. To combat this pro-aging effect, eat a handful of peanuts or roasted soybeans after working out.

As much as we want to *encourage* food that is rich in antioxidants, we want to *discourage* foods that are pro-oxidative and that interfere with key metabolic processes. These foods can be summed up in a phrase: processed foods. Manufactured foods that are baked and fried tend to be rich in the reconfigured oils known as partially hydrogenated oils. These include most fried foods sold in restaurants, most bakery goods but especially doughnuts, cookies, and cake mixes, piecrusts, snack foods such as potato chips and crackers, and other prepared and packaged foods containing coconut, palm, and cottonseed oils. Even hydrogenated polyunsaturated oils such as corn and safflower have to be avoided because they are highly reactive and produce pro-aging free radicals quickly. The best fats for cooking are olive and canola oils.

Flaxseed oil and Brazil nuts are excellent sources of essential fatty acids, which brain cells need to function properly. About one or two tablespoonfuls a day or six to twelve nuts fulfill some of the dietary requirement. Look for "high-lignin" flaxseed oil that is "MAP processed."

Throw away your margarine, which is a particularly virulent promoter of the sludging of your metabolic system. Margarine is known as a *trans-fatty acid*, which plays havoc with the normal functioning of your cells. A Harvard study found that women who ate only four teaspoons of margarine a day had a two-thirds higher risk of heart disease than those eating almost none.

The basic Antiaging Cocktail (page 91) includes antioxidant supplements, but a good deal of evidence supports the conclusion that the body utilizes antioxidants best in foods, which are nature's vehicles for delivering valuable nutrients in the best possible combination for your body. The colorful fruits (berries, citrus, red and purple grapes, tomatoes) and dark green vegetables (spinach, broccoli, cabbage, kale) are excellent sources of these antiaging nutrients. The more naturally colorful your meal is, the more likely you are to get valuable phytonutrients (plant nutrients) that are antiaging and can protect you from cancer.

One last note: Coffee is not a big issue for those low in acetylcholine. In fact, the caffeine in coffee can actually assist in the stimulation of some cognitive abilities. But the downside is that caffeine in more than moderate doses has other bad effects, including accentuating gastric acid secretion and ulcers, and can lead to insulin and blood sugar imbalances.

If tea isn't part of your regular diet, make a point of including it. The leaves of the plant *Camellia sinensis,* what we know as "tea," are filled with natural antioxidants. Numerous studies have indicated that their large consumption of tea is an important factor in the Japanese and Chinese having a much lower incidence of cancer than Western cultures. Similarly, a recent Norwegian study of twenty thousand people revealed that those who drank just one cup of tea daily had significantly longer life spans. An Italian study showed that drinking a cup of tea daily stimulates antioxidant activity in your blood by 50 percent. Almost any type of green (Japanese), white, or black tea, which even includes good old Lipton's in a bag, will do. Other herbal tea beverages, which do not contain *Camellia sinensis,* lack its antioxidant punch but may have other beneficial properties.

The more variety you have in your diet, the greater chance of getting the nutrients your body needs. Surveys indicate that the average person has a very set and narrow pattern of eating, which becomes more entrenched as you get older. As a result, you can develop deficiencies that may take years to express themselves as a disease. Eating a wide range of foods—ethnic foods combined with traditional American fare—can be stimulating to your brain and body.

Sample Menu

Below is a sample daily menu rich in mind-enhancing nutrients. You can find other recommended Mind Pathway–appropriate foods in chapter 17. We'll talk about your caloric needs once you calculate in your Energy Factor in chapter 11. Use these recommendations as the foundation for your diet.

BREAKFAST

Oat-based cereal or cooked non-instant oatmeal with nonfat milk or soy milk, sprinkled with ¹/₈ teaspoon of cinnamon and a generous helping of fresh refrigerated wheat germ

$^1/_2$ red grapefruit
Fresh cup of coffee or green or black tea

MID-MORNING SNACK
Handful of unsalted, dry-roasted peanuts and seeds mixed with
some dry-roasted soybeans

LUNCH
3–6-ounce grilled swordfish fillet or very lean cut of naturally
raised (hormone-free, non–force-fed, free-range) beef
Mediterranean-type salad with avocado, garbanzo beans, green
beans, tomato, onion, bean sprouts, red bell pepper, and an
olive oil and lemon dressing
Cup of fresh berries
Glass of iced black or green tea, cranberry juice, or soy-based drink

AFTERNOON SNACK
Small bag of trail mix with raisins, almonds, Brazil nuts, soybeans,
and pecans
Cup of coffee (if necessary), black tea, or soy milk
or,
"Super Choline Shake": fresh or frozen berries, juice, and 1 teaspoon of honey, 1–2 teaspoons of lemon or lime juice, and a
sprinkle of brewer's yeast, plus 5 grams or more of high grade
lecithen, containing 95% phosphatidyl choline

DINNER
Split pea soup spiced with turmeric and fresh cracked pepper
Spinach salad with lentils, garbanzo beans, bean sprouts, broccoli,
and $^1/_2$ cooked egg yolk sprinkled with slivered almonds
Garlic-lemon chicken ($^1/_4$ chicken)
Side of whipped sweet potato or squash
Cup of green or black tea, such as oolong or Earl Grey

Regimen Recap

Supplements

Modify the Antiaging Cocktail as follows:

- Mitochondrial protectors: Increase to: CoQ10, 100 mg; acetyl L-carnitine, 500 mg; alpha lipoic acid, 100 mg.
- Antioxidant supplements: Boost all to mid-range.
- B vitamins: Take all twice daily at recommended levels except increase B_1 to 3–8 grams daily and increase B_{12} to 500–1,000 mg twice daily.
- Herbs and spices: Increase gingko biloba to 40 mg three times daily.
- Smart oils: Increase flaxseed or fish oil to 2 tablespoons daily.

Add these new supplements:

- Phosphatidylserine, 100 mg, two to three times daily.
- Ibuprofen, 200–600 mg (200 mg one to three times daily if no stomach or ulcer problems).
- Lecithin (90 percent phosphatidylcholine), 15–30 grams (5–10 mg) three times daily with food; stop lecithin if not better in two to six weeks.
- DMAE bitartrate, 100–1,000 mg.

Pharmaceuticals

If you are a Mind Pathway type whose score is greater than 30, consult with your doctor about these prescription medications: Selegiline (also brand named Deprenyl or Eldepryl), sex hormones (testosterone and/or estrogen), Piracetam, Lucidril (also known as centrophenoxine), and Vinpocetine.

Exercise

Mind-body coordination: one hour twice a week of one or a combination of the following: tai chi, tae kwan do, or other martial arts; tennis; volleyball; badminton.

Diet

◆ Eat foods rich in vitamin B complex, antioxidants, essential fatty acids, and choline.

◆ Drink black or green tea.

◆ Avoid packaged and fried foods.

◆ Avoid margarine.

◆ Avoid foods with saturated fats (meats, whole milk, cheese).

Mind Pathway Case Study

"Arthur Doesn't Seem Himself"

Arthur, a dentist in his mid-fifties, had no intention of coming to our clinic. He wasn't even aware that anything was wrong with him. But his wife was. She couldn't quite put her finger on it, but she knew something was wrong.

"He's just different, Doctor. At first I thought it was my imagination. But gradually I noticed he was becoming more forgetful, couldn't remember where he put his keys, and forgot the dinner plans with friends that we had talked about that very morning. He's a little more irritable and, to be quite frank, less interested in me," she said. Occasionally, he would also forget directions and appear disoriented.

When Arthur arrived at the clinic, he was pleasant enough but thought the visit was a bit silly. "There's nothing wrong with me except maybe a few extra pounds. I'm here only because my wife insisted," he said. He reluctantly took the Mind-Body-Spirit Quotient, and his test results indicated that there was something exceedingly wrong. His test scores on the Mind questionnaire were very high—red flag number one, indicating executive function of his brain and his acetylcholine system were impaired. Because his score was so high, we ordered additional tests, including a PET scan (positron emission tomography) and an apolipoprotein genetic profile blood test. The blood test hinted that Arthur might have a genetic predisposition

Not all fats are equal. Avoid shortening and margarine as well as corn, safflower, and sunflower oils. These polyunsaturated fats are very easily oxidized, thereby forming and releasing free radicals and promoting accelerated aging.

toward Alzheimer's disease. There were abnormal changes in the blood test, suggesting that Arthur had a slightly greater than average risk for Alzheimer's disease. The PET brain scan revealed some mild abnormalities of metabolism in the areas of the brain where Alzheimer's disease mostly occurs.

As a health care professional, he knew to eat a healthy diet low in polyunsaturated fats and refined carbohydrates and ate plenty of fruits and dark, leafy green vegetables (although he had a weakness for canned soda pop—as many as eight cans per day!). In the kitchen, Arthur and his wife liked to use their favorite old aluminum pots for cooking. When we asked about his medications, he said that he was "clear" in that department. "The only thing I take is a daily vitamin pill with extra iron and a couple of teaspoons of Geritol—you know, to keep my red blood cells strong as I get older." Red flag number two.

To replenish his acetylcholine system, a cause of his diminished cognitive abilities, Arthur was placed on a regimen of smart *nutriceuticals* (nutrients and supplements having druglike effects) based on the Antiaging Cocktail but modified to include 1 gram of ALC upon waking, which was slowly increased to a daily total of 2 grams over several weeks; B_1, gradually increased to a daily total of 4 to 6 grams; B_{12}, boosted to 2,000 micrograms daily; and the rest of the B vitamins in the Antiaging Cocktail increased to the mid to high range and twice daily. Added to the regimen was 100 milligrams of phosphatidylserine, three times daily. I made sure he was not on any anticoagulant drugs, which could have a negative effect when taken with the phosphatidylserine. Four weeks later I gave him a trial dose of 400 milligrams of DMAE to determine the status of his acetylcholine-producing system. Three weeks later, Arthur was better, and the DMAE was continued and increased as tolerated.

> **Great Mind Pathway snack foods are pumpkin and other seeds rich in choline. Likewise, season food with sesame seeds.**

Because his tests had revealed a predisposition to Alzheimer's, we instructed him to use antiinflammatory agents like Ibuprofen for muscle and joint aches and pains, as long as he did not have stomach or other intestinal ulcers or kidney problems. (Antiinflammatory agents, other than aspirin, have been shown to decrease the chances of full-blown Alzheimer's dementia.) And to boost blood flow into and throughout the brain, he was told to take 40 milligrams of ginkgo biloba three times a day.

Arthur was immediately taken off Geritol, and his habit of slugging back cans of soda pop all day was halted. Predisposed to a Mind Pathway aging track, Arthur was making matters worse by digging himself into a pro-oxidative and a pro-aging hole by inadvertently increasing his exposure to iron and aluminum. The notion that all old people need more iron than normal in their blood is a myth—and a dangerous one at that. Too many metallic minerals (especially iron, aluminum, copper, and manganese, and, of course, the heavy metals known to be toxic) can have a pro-oxidative/aging effect when they build up and become stored in excess.

Over the years, through his daily spoonful of Geritol and his exposure to aluminum in soda pop cans and cookware, Arthur's levels of iron and aluminum had become exceedingly high. The aluminum was tying up and displacing the other good minerals needed for his own natural antioxidant forces to function and be effective. This allowed the free radicals to run havoc through his body and caused the acceleration of the aging process.

With free radicals surging through him, Arthur needed to flood his body with a diet rich in antioxidants. He began eating plenty of dark-meat ocean fish (salmon, mackerel, sardines, tuna), dark green vegetables, lots of berries and red grapes, and he used olive oil in place of other cooking oils, and butter instead of margarine. He also began drinking a cup of antioxidant-rich green tea with breakfast and dinner instead of his usual coffee, which he limited to midday. We switched him from whole dairy milk to soy milk, the soybean being perhaps the most potent and diverse natural source of many antiaging nutrients and a memory booster as well.

Arthur was beginning to suffer some oxidative damage to his brain. His career was more rote than stimulating, so to help restore the plasticity of his thinking process, we encouraged Arthur to take up games of skill, memory, and strategy. "Well, that's all my wife needed to hear. She finally got me to start playing bridge," he related to us at his first monthly checkup.

Our exercise strategy for Arthur also extended to the physical. On weekends he began playing doubles tennis again, a sport that involves a good deal of planning and memory skills. During the week he would join others in his local park for a morning tai chi martial arts class held every other day. Martial arts in general, but tai chi in particular, require mind-stimulating coordination and concentration.

To rekindle the interest in each other, Arthur and his wife were encouraged to enroll in a White Tantra yoga class. White Tantra is a nonsexual couples yoga in which, through coupled breathing and nonsexual touching, partners begin to enjoy each other in new ways. It also encourages exploration of mutual sound vibrations and sound harmonies which affect the brain via subtle energy systems that promote healing and harmony, and awaken dormant energy centers known as the chakras.

After six months on this regimen, Arthur was returning to his old self, but in a slightly improved version. His memory was enhanced, and he felt more "grounded" in general. "He doesn't stare off into the distance anymore," his wife said. "She's just mad because I'm beating her at bridge," he retorted. As an added benefit to his pro-longevity, mind-enhanced diet and exercise regimen, he had shed twenty pounds.

Because he has a Mind Pathway predilection to Alzheimer's disease, we will be especially alert to any deterioration in Arthur's cognitive abilities and adjust his regimen as needed. Eventually, he may need testosterone replacement therapy. (If Arthur were a woman, "she" would need estrogen replacement therapy.) Inadequate supplies of either can cause memory loss. But for now, Arthur is back on an antiaging track.

9

Body Pathway

Most aging results in a neurotransmitter imbalance rather than a depletion of all the neurotransmitters. A deficiency in a main neurotransmitter results in the entire neural network becoming dysfunctional.

If you have a Body Pathway aging profile, chances are you have a deficiency in dopamine. Like Mind Pathway types, your brain levels of serotonin are just fine, but because your dopamine brain levels are low, your serotonin levels have a more pronounced effect. As you will recall, serotonin acts as an inhibitory neurotransmitter that regulates your sleeping cycle and has a calming influence on the brain and behavior. When serotonin supplies run wild and dopamine supplies are depleted, Body Pathway types feel de-energized. They are passive and less alert. They experience a decreased interest in work, relationships, and life in general. They're *too* calm.

Mind Pathway and Body Pathway types are similar in another way: Both produce excitatory neurotransmitters—the opposite of the serotonin (Spirit Pathway) nervous system, which is governed by inhibitory neurotransmitters. While the acetylcholine and dopamine neurotransmitters have different chemical structures, and in most cases different functions, they are both vital to libido—our sexual drive and the sexual experience. They are both used by the limbic or primitive part of our brains that rule our physical drives and emotions, including sex. Too little of either neurotransmitter, and we lose interest in sex and lose the wide variety of pleasurable sexual sensations and their memories.

If the acetylcholine system governs the so-called higher mental functions (learning, memory, long-term planning, and processing information), the qualities that most define humans as a species, the dopamine system reminds us that we're also animals with basic animal needs. Dopamine is responsible for many of the important body functions: initiation of movement (being able to move quickly from sitting to standing and to change directions); instinctual, spontaneous movements and reactions; muscle tone; posture; addiction to stimulants; hunger; and sex drive. It opens the lungs' airways, regulates pleasure, and influences aggressive behavior.

Primitive Animal Drives

Lacking primitive animal drives and survival instincts to some degree, individuals on the Body Pathway aging track have a tendency to be classically passive-aggressive. They will manipulate you with words and language, but will never take physical action against you. They will never rage, hit you, or break down doors, but they will pound you verbally. They are the brainy, lethargic types; they don't have the energy to do physical exercise, but they never run out of energy to talk up a storm. Think of the characters portrayed by Woody Allen in his films. If Mind Pathway types tend sometimes to be oblivious to what ails them and to the world in general, Body Pathway types are acutely aware of themselves and the world 'around them. They are voracious readers and news junkies.

Body Pathway types tend to complain of weariness and physical fatigue but have a high mental energy. Their depleted dopamine supplies make them candidates for infectious diseases; this type does not feel like being physically active, which can lead to immune decline and a depressed mood. As they age, they develop increasing stiffness and loss of mobility, resulting in biomechanical dysfunction, including stiff joints, poor postural and balance reflexes, and a diminished breathing capacity. When they walk or move, there is a lack of normal arm swing.

Body Pathway types not only feel more tired but *look* more

tired. Their depleted supply of dopamine results in decreased facial expression. Smiling can be a chore.

Their self-awareness often makes them bright and inquisitive people, but the downside is that their inward perspective just as often makes them loners. They literally prefer their own company; socializing is just too tiring.

The feeling of helplessness that Body Pathway types experience is also a consequence of their depleted supply of dopamine and may explain their tendency to depression. In an experiment to test this theory, rats were plunged into cold water, which depleted their dopamine supply, and then placed in a pen where a mild electrical shock was administered. They could easily escape the discomfort by jumping over a small barrier to a shock-free area. Rats who were plunged into warm water for the same time (their dopamine supplies undiminished) jumped to safety from the electric zone. The dopamine-depleted rats just sat there and shivered. The experiment was repeated by inducing dopamine depletion with a chemical compound, and the same result was obtained. The dopamine-depleted rats were paralyzed by inertia.

Avoid all deep-fried foods. Stir-fried foods are okay if a "good" oil (canola, or olive) is added at the end of cooking and is not burned. (When the oil burns, it forms substances that promote free radicals, and it interferes with normal metabolism.) Store all oils and fats in your refrigerator. Heat and light can make oils rancid.

Physiologically, the most extreme depletion of dopamine results in Parkinson's disease, which is characterized by a loss of motor control, notably an uncontrollable resting tremor, rigidity, slowness of movement, and a lack of expressive movements. Often there is a stiff, stooped posture classically accompanied by a shuffling gait and a lack of facial expression. There are poor postural reflexes, which can lead to frequent falls. About one-third of Parkinson's patients go on to develop Alzheimer's disease.

It has been theorized that idiopathic Parkinson's disease ("idiopathic" means the cause is not clear) is in part the result of oxidative damage to the dopamine-producing nerve cells of the brain. The dopamine neurons are very susceptible to "auto-oxidation," meaning the normal release of dopamine leads to the production of hydroxyl-free radicals, which are toxic to the dopamine nerve cell itself and neighboring cells. Some sufferers of Parkinson's do respond positively to large doses of broad-spectrum antioxidant therapy, which included both the fat- and water-soluble antioxidant groups.

There is one other important function of the dopamine system that declines with age, but especially for those on a Body Pathway. Dopamine releases growth hormone from the pituitary gland. As discussed in chapter 5, GH is important in many ways. It is the only strategy available that has the potential to increase nerve growth factors overall in the brain by way of nerve cell regeneration.

A possible downside of GH use is that it affects the whole brain and not just the dopamine system. That can be a plus, however, because if the Body Pathway person goes on to develop Parkinson's, then often many different brain regions are affected. They may already be subtly injured in the silent preclinical state that we call aging. Growth hormone could be protective and regenerative. There are many clinical trials in progress that are examining the use of growth hormone and its family of compounds for the treatment of severe neurodegenerative diseases such as ALS (Lou Gehrig's disease), Alzheimer's, and other conditions.

Your Antiaging Regimen

Supplements

All of us suffer a decline in the dopamine neurotransmitters with aging. Body Pathway types have a pronounced decline. Does that mean they will necessarily get Parkinson's? No. To date, however, there is no way of predicting, and, unfortunately, about 70 to 80 percent of the dopamine neurons are lost before a person starts to show obvious clinical signs of Parkinson's. In other words, by the time you can see or feel the classic signs and symptoms of Parkinson's, the damage is largely irreversible. Body Pathway antiaging strategies are targeted to preserving and protecting the 10 million or so dopamine-producing nerve cells, which in the scheme of the body's several trillion cells are a precious commodity.

Since the Body Pathway aging track is largely caused by environmental and lifestyle rather than genetic factors, our first line of defense is the antioxidant supplements recommended in the Antiaging Cocktail on page 101 that combat free radicals. These include vitamin C and the plant antioxidant flavonoids, vitamin E, CoQ10, alpha lipoic acid, and the carotenoids. A supporting cast of minerals and trace metals activate the antioxidant systems.

The brain's dopamine system is especially vulnerable to free radical damage, partly because of a self-destructive process. As the dopamine brain cells are transformed into their metabolic by-product called norepinephrine, they release an especially toxic form of free radicals that damage healthy dopamine cells. In this sense, the dopamine system helps to sow the seeds of its own destruction.

The second antiaging defense strategy is to provide additional supplies from which to make more dopamine. The amino acid tyrosine, by making more dopamine, has a stimulating effect that counteracts the tendency of Body Pathway types to be lethargic, negative, and slightly depressed.

L-tyrosine is available as an over-the-counter supplement at most health stores. Depending on your individual physiology, take between 50 and 500 milligrams, always on an empty stomach. Build the dosage gradually until you find a level that is effective for you. Remember the first rule of antiaging supplements: *Start low and go slow.* The undesired side effects of tyrosine in high doses can be overstimulation, excitement, loss of appetite, or a change in blood pressure. It seems to be most effective in getting into the brain nerve cells and producing results after the nerve cells have been firing or working the most and are the most depleted, such as from physical or mental stress.

The two-hour window immediately following weight training is when muscles are most receptive to rebuilding. Maximize your weight-resistance exercise with a drink rich in whey or casein protein, soy isolate protein, or vegetable protein.

An alternative to tyrosine is the related amino acid phenylalanine, also a building block for the manufacture of dopamine and norepinephrine. While both amino acids have the same essential function, some people have a marked preference for tyrosine or phenylalanine. (My experience indicates that most patients do better with tyrosine.) There are two forms of phenylalanine, D and L, and a mixture of both is called DLPA. Take amino acids before the afternoon since they can cause insomnia. *Note:* Phenylalanine and tyrosine need folic acid, vitamins B_3, C, and B_6 to be converted to dopamine, both part of our Antiaging Cocktail discussed in chapter 7.

Caution: Pregnant women should not take phenylalanine, because it can have a very serious negative developmental effect in the brain of the fetus. For the same reason, pregnant women and small children should avoid artificial sweeteners containing aspartame (marketed under the brand names Equal and NutraSweet), which contains phenylalanine. One twelve-ounce can of soda can contain as much as 200 milligrams of aspartame. Persons on antiaging programs should avoid all artificial sweeteners. Phenylalanine is to be avoided if you have high blood pressure, cardiac arrhythmias, or a genetic disorder called phenylketonuria (PKU), a condition where you build up excessive toxic blood levels of phenylalanine. Also avoid tyrosine if you have melanoma or any type of active tumor. Avoid taking these amino acids if you are are on pyschotropic drugs, which can he intensified by tyrosine or phenylalanine.

If dopamine self-generated free radicals weren't bad enough, other types of toxic, free radical molecules also target these sensitive dopamine cells. The most serious attack occurs in structures inside the cell called the mitochondria. The mitochondria are energy factories of the cell where both energy and energy by-products (free-radical pro-oxidants) are produced. Damage to mitochondrial DNA accelerates the aging process of all parts of the body, but certain organs are especially sensitive to this type of damage, including the brain. The brain is quite susceptible to oxidative free-radical damage because it consumes about 20 percent of your total oxygen intake.

It is vital, then, for Body Pathway types to take the mitochondrial protecting agents in the Antiaging Cocktail, including acetyl L-carnitine, alpha lipoic acid, CoQ10, Vitamin E, N-acetyl L-cysteine, plus the "core antioxidants."

All the supplements are available over the counter at most health food stores and from mail order supplement and pharmaceutical suppliers. See the Regimen Recap on page 99 for dosage recommendations. See Antiaging Supplement Suppliers in the appendix for items not available at your local drugstore.

Pharmaceuticals

If you rated a high score of 20 points or more on the Body part of your Mind-Body-Spirit Quotient, you should consider consulting a knowledgeable health care professional about taking pro–Body

Pathway medications. Elderyl, also known as Deprenyl (selegiline is the scientific name), may retard the degeneration of the very sensitive dopamine-producing neurons. Some consider it to have neuroprotective properties because it inhibits the oxidation of dopamine. Bromocriptine can be used to accentuate the effects of existing dopamine supplies or the effects of dopamine precursors. Consult with a knowledgeable medical doctor.

Therapy with the GH family of compounds can be especially beneficial to high-scoring Body Pathway types, leading to increased levels of a growth factor called IGF-1 and other growth factors in the brain and spinal fluid. The IGF-1 factor, combined with the direct effects of growth hormone itself on nerve cells, energizes and revitalizes the brain and the whole body. The Body Pathway type can benefit because GH can also interfere with the programmed cell death process called apoptosis.

GH is available only with a doctor's prescription and comes in an injectable form. Several major pharmaceutical manufacturers have ongoing human trials with oral tablets that stimulate growth hormone release. These appear safe in early trials.

Men may also consider consulting their physician about testosterone replacement therapy. Many of the symptoms of a declining dopamine-norepinephrine supply—loss of libido and sex drive, diminished energy, poor mood and muscularity—could simply be the result of a deficiency in testosterone. More on this in chapter 12, Your Sex Factor.

Exercise

In our Mind-Body-Spirit paradigm in chapter 7, the dopamine neurotransmitter system was identified as the Body Pathway element. It governs our primitive, physical side of being a human being, including the ability to move normally (locomotion). Too little dopamine results in lack of initiative and decreased physical activity. Many athletes and weight lifters take dopamine-like stimulants, such as caffeine, Ma Huang herb, guarana herb, and ephedrine, to get a more powerful workout from increased motivation and drive. Body Pathway persons can overstimulate their systems with these stimulants, speeding up the aging auto-oxidation and degeneration of this system.

Body Pathway types may have a high fat-to-muscle ratio. Think
flab—not a pretty picture. But there is more to decreasing
flab than just looking good. An underused musculature can begin a downward spiral of diminished
breathing capacity, creaky joints, increased incidence of injuries, and a general decline in the
body's biomechanical system with a profound
pro-aging result.

Deeply and richly
colored fruits and vegetables
are the highest in antioxidants
and phytonutrients. If your meal
doesn't include fresh (raw, uncooked)
food items with naturally brilliant
colors, you are not eating in
antiaging style. Think
natural color!

The goal of the Body Pathway exercise
regimen is to minimize the negative effects of a
depleted dopamine system through a multilevel
program of stretching muscles and developing
muscle mass; enhancing posture, balance, and coordination; developing spatial orientation; and increasing reaction time.
The hands-on manipulation of the soft tissues (muscles, tendons,
and the body's connective tissue envelope called the myofascia),
using deep tissue massage techniques, is encouraged to release tight
structures and make movements more fluid.

To facilitate postural reflexes, reaction time, and coordination,
both the Feldenkreis and the Alexander Method are effective.
Feldenkreis teaches awareness through movement using mental
and physical training methods utilizing mental imagery coupled
with the exploration of new movement patterns. The Alexander
Method uses light touching and massage to realign posture and create awareness of movement in space.

Yoga is also an important element of the Body Pathway exercise
regimen. Use hatha and other yoga methods to stretch out tight
muscles and tissues. Kundalini and tantra yoga can increase breathing capacity and spinal alignment, and stimulate sexual and other
energy centers (or "chakras," in yogic terms).

To build muscle mass, begin a weight-training program. If
you've never used weights before, consult a professionally licensed
personal trainer. Here are some basic rules of thumb we use at our
Sports Medicine and Anti-Aging Medical Group in Santa Monica,
California:

◆ Do not weight-train for more than thirty or forty minutes
   in one day; otherwise, you can overtrain and cause a decline
   in your natural anabolic hormones. That will defeat the pur-

pose of your program and increase oxidative (free radical) stress.

◆ Do not use weights more than two days in a row. Continuous daily training can slow down the muscle-building process.

◆ Always begin your weight-training session with twenty minutes or so of aerobic exercise (enough to get you sweating) so that when the weights are started, your tissues will be warm and pliable and less likely to be injured.

◆ Do two sets of each type of weight-resistance exercise. In the first set, do twelve to fifteen repetitions. In the second set do six to eight repetitions with an increased weight. When you are at the last two to three repetitions, you should have a muscle "failure" or inability to do more. If you don't, then the weight needs to be increased. The total number of sets per training session should be limited to a maximum of nine to twelve. To build maximum muscle mass, vary the types of repetitions between workouts. Alternately, begin the first set with the highest weight and then follow the remaining sets with decreased weights.

◆ Identify your starting lift (first-set weight) with the one-lift maximum test: Find the maximum weight you can lift only once; slowly work up to it. Start with a light weight and work up to the maximum weight, or have your trainer assist you with the help of a chart that can determine your maximum one lift. Then start by using a weight that is 60 to 70 percent of that maximum weight. That is the starting weight for your first set. Example: If you can lift only forty pounds once and no more, then your initial lift weight is about twenty-five to thirty pounds.

◆ Increase your initial weight until you can do six or eight repetitions. That's your second set lift.

◆ After two sets, move on to the next weight resistance exercise.

◆ After a weight-training session, stretch out the areas just exercised and any other tight muscles for at least forty-five seconds to 1 minute per stretch. A stretch doesn't work unless it is held at least that long.

Diet

We want to build a diet plan rich in foods that are high in tyrosine and phenylalanine, the amino acids that are used by dopamine. At the same time, we don't want to include a lot of foods that will increase a feeling of lethargy, which means avoiding pure carbohydrates, or starches (potatoes, yams, corn and carrots). Ideal are protein-rich foods that are high in tyrosine/phenylalanine and low in the competitor amino acid tryptophan that can make you slow down.

Fortunately, many high-protein foods are excellent sources of tyrosine, including chicken and turkey breast, low-fat or nonfat cottage cheese, yogurt, tuna, eggs, and seafood such as swordfish, red snapper, salmon, and shrimp. For vegetarians, choose tofu, beans, peas, lentils, and soybeans, including soybean-based veggieburgers and the like.

A number of vitamins and minerals are especially good at helping in the synthesis of dopamine from tyrosine, including the B vitamins, folic acid, vitamin C, and minerals. Foods rich in B vitamins tend to be rich in tyrosine as well, including fish and dairy products. Vitamin C can be found in the colorful fruits and vegetables, which are also great sources of antioxidants. But to maximize the Body Pathway diet, separate the consumption of pure carbohydrates (such as fruits and vegetables) from the proteins. Try to eat the carbohydrates one to two hours after your high-protein food or at night to help you sleep.

Magnesium is particularly interesting for the Body Pathway aging track. Magnesium helps to lower free-radical activity; by enhancing blood flow to the brain, it reduces blood vessel spasm. It also protects the cell's mitochondria, one of our main antiaging strategies for Body Pathway types. Alarmingly, it is estimated that only one in four Americans get the minimum amount of magnesium needed by the body. Foods rich in magnesium include whole grains, nuts (especially almonds), seeds (pumpkin and squash), and legumes (especially soybeans and lima beans). Bran cereal and oatmeal are also excellent sources of magnesium, but, again, limit their intake because they are almost pure carbohydrate.

For additional antioxidant phytonutrient boosting, season your food with plenty of garlic, turmeric (curry powder), fresh parsley, onions and pepper, including cayenne, chili pepper, and freshly cracked black pepper. See the Antiaging Cocktail in chapter 7 for more on this.

Avoid foods that are pro-oxidative, including many processed and packaged foods made with polyunsaturated fats and partially hydrogenated fats, especially those containing corn and safflower oils. Among the worst offenders are snack foods (potato chips, corn chips, and so forth), bakery items (cookies, pastries, crackers, doughnuts, and others) sold in packages or at bakeries, popcorn sold at theaters, and most fried fast food.

Tyrosine and phenylalanine are building blocks for the production of dopamine. Foods rich in these amino acids include lean meat, low-fat cheese, nonfat milk, and—hold on to your candy bar— chocolate. (Keep in mind, though, that most chocolate food items are loaded with sugar and fat. Go easy!)

As we've discussed, Body Pathway types tend to feel tired and lackluster because of their depleted supplies of dopamine. Until your dopamine levels have been restored, make a power energy shake if you experience fatigue during the day. Use a supplement powder that contains any of these three main protein sources: egg, milk-derived (whey or casein), or plant (soy or no-soy, including peas and beans). It's your choice; some people cannot tolerate the lactose in the milk-derived products. For others, the soy or other plant protein products might be easier on their digestion. You also have a choice of liquids to mix the powder with, including soy milk and juices (nonsweetened cranberry, blueberry, or straw-berry are excellent antioxidant sources).

If you aren't terribly fatigued, then make a mixture of half pure soy protein isolate and half whey protein. Your daily need for protein is about 1/3 gram per pound of body weight if you are sedentary and up to 1 gram per pound if you are very physically active and trying to build muscle. Whey or other pure protein or tyrosine capsules are good for a quick charge but not for a long-term antiaging strategy for Body Pathway types and in general. Prolonged intake of a diet high in animal protein is not recommended. Animal-based proteins oxidize easier and promote free radicals as well as osteoporosis. For purposes of antiaging and preservation of your dopamine cells, soy and other vegetable protein foods should be the dominant sources of your protein intake.

For a vegetarian antiaging high-tyrosine boost, make a smoothie from a high-quality soybean protein isolate and a naturally diluted, unsweetened, deeply colored berry juice (blueberry, boysenberry, cranberry). These vegetarian protein drinks can be used as a long-term strategy because they contain more favorable nutrients, such as the isoflavones (which have antioxidant effects and other favorable effects on the blood vessels and other organs), than the protein drinks derived from animal sources.

Tea, that is real tea rather than the herbal beverages called herbal teas, contains polyphenol antioxidants. Black tea is good for Body Pathway types who feel tired to begin with, but don't deny yourself that mid-morning or mid-afternoon cup if it gets you through the day.

To recap, choose your protein sources from foods rich in tyrosine and phenylalanine, preferably from seafood or vegetable protein sources. Space your carbohydrate intake away from the tyrosine-rich proteins and generally decrease or eliminate the starchy carbohydrates that lack antioxidants (such as French fries, pasta, and cookies). Choose from fruits and vegetables rich in antioxidants. Include the B-vitamin-rich foods and the vitamin C foods and breads rich in whole grains, oatmeal bran, and wheat germ. Magnesium-rich almonds and sunflower seeds are a great snack food for Body Pathway types. Avoid pro-oxidative foods rich in harmful corn and safflower oils, including snack foods, bakery, and fried fast food.

Below is a sample daily menu designed especially for the Body Pathway aging track. Amounts will vary according to your body-mass index, which you can discover by taking the test on page 87. Build your own weekly menu by consulting the food index on pages 259–63.

Sample Menu

BREAKFAST
Fruit smoothie: Blend of red or purple grapes, kiwi, strawberries or
    raspberries, and soy milk or nonfat milk.
Low-fat or nonfat cottage cheese (for protein)
Green or black tea

MID-MORNING SNACK
Handful of almonds or roasted soybeans
Cup of coffee or, preferably, green or black tea with a slice of lemon

LUNCH

Turkey breast or veggieburger sandwich on whole-grain bread (no mayonnaise)

Garden salad with spinach, red or yellow bell peppers, broccoli, onion, cauliflower, and beets with a fresh Italian dressing containing olive oil, garlic, and freshly cracked pepper

Soy chocolate pudding (2 ounces of silken tofu mixed with 1 tablespoon of honey and 2 to 3 tablespoons of cocoa powder; blend and chill before eating)

AFTERNOON SNACK

Red or purple grapes or unsweetened concord grape juice

DINNER

Gazpacho

Chilean sea bass sautéed lightly in canola oil and seasoned with lemon and garlic

Side of lima beans seasoned with turmeric or cayenne pepper

Cup of frozen vanilla yogurt on fresh fruit (such as melon or berries)

Cup of hot black or green tea

Regimen Recap

Supplements

Modify the Antiaging Cocktail with the following:

◆ Antioxidant supplements: Increase to the upper range except vitamin A; delete copper
◆ Mitochondrial protectors: Increase CoQ10, 100 mg; acetyl L-carnitine, 500 mg; alpha lipoic acid, 250–500 mg
◆ B vitamins: Take all twice daily; start B_{12} at mid-range and increase as needed
◆ Herbs and spices: Increase garlic, parsley, turmeric, pepper and ginkgo biloba

Add these new supplements:

- Tyrosine (L-tyrosine), 50–500 mg as needed, two to three times daily between meals on an empty stomach
  or,
- Phenylalanine (L-phenylaline), 50–500 mg as needed, two to three times daily between meals on an empty stomach

Medications (prescription only)

- Increase selegiline or bromocriptine or other dopamine agonists under doctor's supervision.

Exercise

- Posture, balance, and coordination: Feldenkreis or Alexander Method, once a week
- Stretching of muscles and tissues: yoga, fifteen minutes per day
- Muscle mass: Weight-resistance training, three times a week, every other day
- Light to moderate intensity walking or bicycling

Diet

- This is a high-protein, low-carbohydrate diet; eat the proteins before the carbohydrates.
- Keep fat intake low when eating protein; avoid fried foods.
- Select protein from foods rich in tyrosine/phenylalanine.
- Select low-glycemic fruits (which raise blood sugar levels slowly) and deeply colored vegetables rich in antioxidants and phytonutrients.
- Include foods rich in magnesium.
- Season food with spices rich in antioxidant phytonutrients.
- Avoid snack foods, bakery, fried fast food, and other foods loaded with pro-oxidative polyunsaturated and partially hydrogenated fats and oils.
- Avoid dark meats from animals, which can be a source of iron.
- Avoid iron intake unless you are being treated for an iron-deficient medical condition.

Body Pathway Case Study

"Bob Wakes Up"

"I feel as if I'm sleepwalking all the time. I'm tired when I get up, in the afternoon, and at night," said Bob during his initial visit to the Sports Medicine and Anti-Aging Medical Group in Santa Monica, California. There was no doubt that Bob was telling the truth. He even *looked* tired. He was stooped forward and shuffled when he walked. Even getting up on the examining table was an effort. All this in an ostensibly healthy man who had just seen his fortieth birthday.

"But it's more than that," Bob continued. "I feel as though I'm in a fog. It's starting to affect my work." Bob is a creative advertising executive whose work depends on a certain amount of business-related socializing. Once a self-described party animal, he just didn't have the energy anymore to network at industry parties, much less the golf course.

Divorced, Bob had been engaged and was to get married two years ago, but he finally abandoned the whole idea. "Between the wedding and honeymoon plans and moving our separate households together, well, I loved her, but it was too much. I just didn't have the energy," he said.

His score on the Mind-Body-Spirit Quotient indicated a deficiency in the dopamine system. In addition to being chronically fatigued, his Lifestyle Factor score indicated he was mildly depressed and socially isolated. He also had some family history of Parkinson's disease, the most extreme expression of the Body Pathway aging track. We dug a little deeper to find out what kind of help Bob had been getting.

A well-read guy who was up on the latest health trends, Bob had created a multilevel regimen for himself to fix his fatigue problem. He ate plenty of carbohydrates for energy, took melatonin at night to help him sleep, and jogged or biked to keep himself trim— that is, whenever he had the energy. He occasionally took Prozac to get his spirits up when he was feeling especially blue.

Nice regimen, wrong person.

Bob was, in fact, exacerbating his existing dopamine deficiency with his self-styled program. We immediately took him off his carbohydrate-loaded diet, which was slowing him down further, and replaced it with a diet rich in protein sources. It contained tyrosine, such as turkey breast, dark-meat fish, peas, beans, tofu and other soy products, lentils, and textured vegetable protein. We taught Bob not only what to eat but also when to eat what. He ate his tyrosine-rich foods first (two hours after his last meal) and waited, if possible, one hour to eat fats or carbohydrates. If this was not possible, then Bob would always eat his low-fat protein first and then finish the meal with low-glycemic vegetables and fruits.

He began eating lots of berries and other deeply colored fruits and vegetables, loaded with antioxidants. When he was feeling especially fatigued—for Bob it was usually in the afternoon—he made a whey or soy protein shake by mixing or blending one scoop of each in a glass of nonfat cow's milk or soy milk. If this was inconvenient, he would take a 500-milligram capsule of L-tyrosine.

His dosage of melatonin was reduced, and his Prozac was eliminated by gradually reducing doses over three weeks. The Prozac and melatonin were pumping up his serotonin effect, and the last thing Bob needed was to increase the levels or action of serotonin, a neurotransmitter that induces a calming effect. His depleted supply of dopamine had already made his serotonin system too dominant.

Instead, Bob was prescribed a regimen of supplements designed to boost his dopamine levels, stimulate his libido and mental faculties, and lubricate his rusty biomechanical system—his muscles, tendons, and joints. Because his dopamine supply was extremely low, I started him on a test dose of the pharmaceutical Eldepryl (Deprenyl), which immediately made him feel more alert and increased his response time to simple tests, such as catching a ball.

To stimulate blood flow to his brain, he took the natural herb ginkgo biloba. His self-described mental fog began to lift. He became more decisive, less irritable, less stressed about his life, and happier.

While Bob was a normal weight for his height (6 feet, 180 pounds) and his Energy Factor indicated he did not have a glucose-metabolism problem, his muscle-to-fat ratio was low because of low blood levels of DHEA and free testosterone. His depleted dopamine levels and his carbohydrate-loaded diet compounded the constant feeling that he was moving in slo-mo. To fight his flab, small doses of DHEA and a moderate dose of L-glutamine, were added to his supplement regimen. He alternated androstenedione with 4-

androstenediol, naturally occurring hormones, two to three times a week to spike his testosterone levels.

He had also been doing the wrong kind of exercise. He was focusing on aerobic exercise (weight loss) rather that anaerobic (muscle gain) exercise. When he tried to run or bike, he was just straining his already tight connective tissue and flabby muscles. Working with a trainer, he began a three-part program that combined a weekly deep-massage technique (he chose a type of Rolfing called Heller Work), a daily fifteen-minute stretch utilizing yoga techniques, a three-times-a-week weight resistance training, and moderate to easy walking and exercise bicycling.

Having never trained with weights before, he was a little apprehensive. But he stuck to the rules of weight training, and never trained more than thirty to forty minutes at one time, alternating rest days with training days that gradually increased his weight resistance, and stretching slowly and deeply after weight training.

A reenergized Bob visited our clinic three months after he started his customized antiaging regimen. He strolled into our office with a new gait and upright posture that spoke of confidence. His handshake was firm, and his face was alert and expressive. He had actually gained a few pounds (muscle weighs more than fat), but his love handles and soft stomach had beaten a fast retreat. He was noticeably more muscular in his upper body and had decreased his body fat by 5 percent.

His social life had improved, too. He was leaving the next day for a long weekend in Cabo San Lucas with a new woman friend. And work? "My work has never been better." he says. "Our agency just landed a huge account—thanks, according to my boss, to my brilliant presentation. Everybody wants to know what I've been taking. I say, you know, a little bit of this, a little bit of that. I may tell them everything later on, but right now I'm enjoying the competitive edge."

~10~

Spirit Pathway

The Spirit Pathway aging profile is a study in excess. Think of Jake La Motta, the main character in Martin Scorsese's classic film, *Raging Bull,* about a serotonin-dysfunctional figure run amok. Spirit Pathway types tend to have poor self-control and are impulse ridden. With the onset of middle age this archetype begins to exhibit more prominently the results of addictive behavior, from overeating and drinking to "superjock" out-of-control athletic endeavors. These are the class overachievers and often make great leaders. Their energy is contagious, and their spontaneity and decisiveness are extremely attractive to all the rest of us who wish we could be so sure of everything.

Because they tend to throw caution to the wind, they are prime candidates for serious health problems derived from lifestyle choices and biochemical imbalances. Much of their behavior is actually a never-ending quest for peace, tranquillity, and comfort caused by their out-of-sync serotonin levels. They are constantly seeking ways to compensate for this hormonal disharmony. They often smoke and drink more than the norm in order to control stress. They also tend to be prone to accidents, depression, and suicidal or high-risk behavior destructive to themselves and others. The injuries sustained to their biomechanical systems and organs (including the brain) earlier in life can have a debilitating effect later, and with age their frequent injuries become much more difficult to heal.

Aging is accelerated by the constant high levels of cortisol in their bloodstream caused by the inability of Spirit Pathway types to *physiologically* buffer stress. They are also at risk of hypertension and damage to brain tissue caused by excessive free-radical production, caused by their compulsive, pro-aging habits, such as alcohol abuse and overeating.

Hyper-hedonistic, Spirit Pathway people can find with age that their sexual performance no longer matches their sexual desire. The accumulated effects of a pro-aging lifestyle lead to decreased blood flow and nerve function of the sex organs.

Spirit Pathway Antiaging Regimen

Supplements

If you are the Jake La Motta aging type, you are probably on edge all the time, yet you are underperforming at work, on the playing field, and in bed. The primary reason is a serotonin imbalance, either because there is a lack of the raw materials that make serotonin, that is, amino acid tryptophan, or there's enough tryptophan but it's not able to enter the brain where serotonin is made.

When insulin works normally and is quickly released after a simple, high-glycemic carbohydrate ingestion, it moves other, non-tryptophan amino acids out of the bloodstream and into the muscles and the liver. No longer competing with these other amino acids, tryptophan easily enters the brain through the protective blood membrane. Once inside the brain, the nerve cell machinery goes to work to make new supplies of serotonin and melatonin. From this new supply the brain levels of serotonin go up, and the "serotonin effect"—a feeling of calm and relaxation—takes hold for up to three hours.

Tryptophan supplements are no longer easily available in the United States. About ten years ago, the Federal Drug Administration pulled tryptophan supplements—or L-tryptophan, as it was known—off the shelves because several people got very sick and some died from a contaminated batch sold by a foreign firm. (The supplement continued to be sold in Europe.) However, a more potent serotonin elevating compound, 5-hydroxytryptophan (5-HTP), has begun to appear in health food stores and mail order catalogs. Although 5-HTP is ten times as potent as L-tryptophan, I prefer the latter. Fewer clinical studies and fewer years of experience (including my own) are available on 5-HTP, and because it converts faster to serotonin, it has the risk of dramatically elevating blood levels of serotonin. And that's not a good idea. Too much serotonin in the bloodstream may damage heart valves, which is the reason Redux was pulled from the market. Unfortunately, L-tryptophan now is only available in the U.S. through compounding pharmacies. Remember, 5-HTP should be used cautiously and for no more than two to three months. In that time, the neurotransmitter imbalance should have been corrected. (L-tryptophan can be taken safely indefinitely.) Redux also worked by elevating serotonin levels. It was eventually found to be associated with damage to heart valves in some patients, which is the primary reason it was pulled from the market.

> Feel a food craving or anxiety attack approaching? A piece of plain white bread can produce a more calming "serotonin effect" than an entire chocolate candy bar.

Twenty-five to fifty milligrams of 5-HTP should be taken between meals (one to two hours before or two to three hours after a meal) or with a pure carbohydrate (French bread, bagel, rice cakes, pretzels, and so forth). The best time to take it is one hour before an early dinner that is eaten no later than 7:00 P.M. No food should be taken after you finish your dinner; ingesting more food will block the effectiveness of 5-HTP. Water or herbal (noncaffeinated) tea are fine. Occasional side effects of 5-HTP have mainly to do with mood. Each individual responds differently, so one person's euphoria or agitation could be another's drowsiness or sleepiness. The maximum daily dose should not exceed 200 milligrams without medical supervision.

Serotonin is the neurotransmitter that the pineal gland uses to make the hormone melatonin. As a regulator of biological rhythms, melatonin is responsible for the body's response to light and dark, or day and night. If you don't produce enough, you literally can't get a good night's sleep (although you may think you are), so during your waking hours, your body is in a constant state of low-level stress. This can be more than just an inconvenience. Stress is also a leading cause of heart disease (the number one killer of men *and* women) and has been linked to cancer and neurodegenerative illnesses such as Parkinson's and Alzheimer's.

Normally, your body produces serotonin throughout the day from your diet, leaving enough for the pineal gland to make melatonin at night. Spirit Pathway types, however, produce such a low level of serotonin that there is no longer any to be made into melatonin. A combination of vitamin B_6, calcium, magnesium, and niacinamide (a form of vitamin B_3) can facilitate the production of serotonin, creating a larger pool from which melatonin can be made.

If you have a serious lack of the serotonin effect in your brain as demonstrated by a high score on the Spirit part of the Mind-Body-Spirit questionnaire on page 85, you may have to temporarily take medicines called selective serotonin reuptake inhibiting drugs, or SSRIs, which include Zoloft, Paxil, and Prozac. These drugs block the reabsorption of serotonin by the nerve cells that make and release it. The overall effect is an increased duration of action but not an increased supply. It may be safer and more natural to use 5-HTP or L-tryptophan to increase the serotonin effect, but an insulin-resistance problem may negate its effect. (See chapter 11 to determine if you have an insulin-resistance problem.)

The older you are, the more likely you are making less melatonin from your serotonin and the more likely your sleep will be fragmented. Sleep is much more than a state of rest. The body uses the down time to release a host of rejuvenating hormones, including the powerful antiaging growth hormone and family of compounds. But if sleep is fragmented, the body never reaches the deep level of sleep during which GH and other important hormones are released. Take a dose of $1/2$ gram of melatonin before bedtime for sleep regulation. Melatonin can also be used in smaller doses to keep the serotonin-melatonin ratios favorable for antiaging effects (even if you don't have a sleeping problem). But don't flood your system with melatonin; as with any hormone, a little goes a long way.

Finally, pregnenolone, a hormone produced in the brain and the adrenal cortex, can also be helpful in stabilizing mood and increasing energy. The hormone declines with age to the point that more than half of its peak supply is lost by age seventy-five.

See Consumer's Guide to Hormone Replacement in the appendix for more information on gender, age and dose recommendations.

Exercise

Spirit Pathway types tend to go through spurts of exercising very intensely, impulsively, and out of control, often injuring themselves. They also embrace exercise trends, trying the latest techniques dispensed by this year's health and fitness guru. Their basements look like exercise equipment graveyards. They have lots of good intentions but little follow-through.

By their biochemistry, Spirit Pathway people are not serene. They're go-getters and risk-takers, which is why we love 'em. However, the last thing they need is a short burst of exercise. That only agitates their minds, which are all over the place anyway.

The core of the Spirit Pathway exercise program is a yogic/meditative activity to cultivate serenity and develop concentration. The goal is to learn self-control and gain inner knowledge of what prompts compulsive behavior, and focus on ways to correct it through thoughts and action.

To keep the cardiovascular and biomechanical systems fit and to balance the serotonin system, a regimen of sixty to ninety minutes of low-intensive exercise (less than 60 percent maximum heart rate), a minimum of three times a week, is recommended. Walking, swimming, and bicycling are good choices.

Spirit Pathway types can be overweight because of the high-caloric foods they prefer and their binge-eating habits. See chapter 11 for tips on fat-burning exercises.

Diet

Because of their naturally compulsive behavior, Spirit Pathway types tend to like foods that alter their moods: alcohol to relax, coffee to stimulate, and rich, fatty foods and foods high in carbohydrates to provide a feeling of comfort. This search for comfort is sometimes mistakenly interpreted by patients as hunger. DHEA can help in this regard, diminishing appetite by synchronizing insulin and glucose levels. Most of my patients who have had a favorable response to DHEA say that it gives them an overall sense of well-being.

To reinforce this effect, Spirit Pathway profilers should be on a "reverse" diet schedule. The "dinner" meal, when the greatest amount of protein is traditionally consumed in the United States, should be eaten *no later* than noon to 2:00 P.M. but optimally earlier. This will stockpile protein energy for the day ahead. Throughout the day the amount of protein is gradually decreased, and the amount of pure carbohydrate (starchy foods like pasta and breads) are increased to enhance the release of serotonin. Eating an evening meal dominated by protein is the worst scenario for Spirit Pathway types, setting the stage for a restless night's sleep.

Meals should be eaten five times daily to avoid the peaks and valleys of moods that can accompany big meals. The idea is not to "graze" but rather to eat five planned and well-timed meals and avoid skipping meals as much as possible.

Use low-calorie/high-carbohydrate meals, of five parts carbohydrates to one part protein when your mood is down or you're getting cravings and needing satisfaction. For Spirit Pathway types, morning meals should have lots of lean protein (egg whites, protein shake). Evening meals should be dominated by starches (pastas, breads, yellow and orange vegetables). After taking your starchy snack (pretzels, French bread, rice cakes, bagels) on an empty stomach, you should start to feel some comfort and less craving within forty-five minutes. If that does not work, then take 25–50 milligrams of 5-HTP capsules or 250–500 milligrams of L-tryptophan.

Beverages with caffeine should be limited to no more than two per day. It makes Spirit Pathway types even more compulsive and can raise insulin and cortisol levels.

Since alcoholic cocktails are pro-aging, we want to limit those as much as possible. It is better to have a glass or two of red wine with dinner—red because the red grape skin is filled with antioxidants that can promote healthy blood vessels and reduce heart disease, which this group is especially prone to.

Studies indicate that 50 percent of those on serotonin-enhancing drugs such as Prozac could benefit by dietary manipulation—the type of food and when it is taken—along with over-the-counter supplements such as 5-HTP or the prescription amino acid L-tryptophan. Below is a typical recommended daily menu designed to pro-

mote the serotonin effect. You can build your own weekly menu of
recommended dishes from choices provided in chapter 17. Choose
the high-tryptophan foods for breakfast and lunch, and gradually
build into a menu of high-glycemic foods for dinner. Use high-
glycemic, non-fatty foods to snack on throughout the day when
cravings strike and to produce a calming effect. Keep in mind
that fats and high fiber retard the serotonin effect you are trying to
achieve.

Sample Menu

BREAKFAST
3-egg omelet (2 whites, 1 whole egg) with fresh herbs and low-fat
    cheese
Half a grapefruit or a sliced kiwi fruit
Cup of coffee (with nonfat dairy creamer)

MID-MORNING SNACK
Trail mix

LUNCH
Salmon or swordfish (3 to 4 ounces) salad with greens, onions and
    a lemon vinaigrette
Baked potato with skin
French bread (no butter)

AFTERNOON SNACK
Carrot sticks or puffed mini rice cakes if craving food or feel agi-
    tated, restless
Tea

DINNER
Pasta primavera
Succotash
Low-fat cheesecake
Herbal (decaffeinated) tea with a tablespoon of honey

Regimen Recap

Supplements

Modify the Antiaging Cocktail as follows:

◆ Increase all the B vitamins by taking them twice daily.
◆ Increase vitamins B_6, B_{12}, and folic acid to a mid-range dose.
◆ Increase vitamin B_3 to 400 mg twice daily.
◆ Increase vitamin B_5 to 250 mg twice daily.
◆ Increase vitamin C to 500–1,000 mg three to four times daily (1 gram at a time).

Add these new supplements:

◆ 5-hydroxytryptophan (5-HTP), 25–200 mg daily; use in 25–100 mg increments as needed between meals or at bedtime or, L-tryptophan: 250–4,000 mg daily; use in 250–500 mg increments
◆ Pregnenolone or DHEA, 5–10 mg in the morning as needed to stabilize mood and increase energy

Exercise

◆ 15 minutes of meditative/stretching type exercise (such as yoga) daily
◆ 60–90 minutes of low-intensity walking or bicycling 3 times a week
◆ 20–30 minutes of resistance weight training every other day

Diet

◆ Use a 70-20-10 protein-carbohydrate-fat/oil ratio in the morning; gradually increase the carbohydrates throughout the day to an inverse ratio of 70-20-10 carbohydrate-protein-fat/oil by the evening.
◆ Five to six meals a day.
◆ Separate carbohydrate intake from proteins and fats/oils by 90 minutes whenever possible.
◆ Snack on starchy foods such as plain French bread or puffed mini rice cakes for food cravings.

Spirit Pathway Case Study

Ms. Jones Loses Control

Ms. Jones came to our clinic with a complaint she can't remember ever *not* having: a weight problem. She had tried all the different diet combinations, from high carbohydrate to low fat to high protein and high fat, ad nauseum. She recognized that her weight problem wasn't entirely the food she ate but how and when she ate. "I'm a binge eater, Doctor. I admit it, so sue me."

A successful talent agent in the entertainment industry, Ms. Jones, forty-four, earned a six-figure salary, ate at the best restaurants on both coasts, and rubbed shoulders with Hollywood's elite. She was also desperate to lose twenty-five to thirty pounds (mostly fat)—no matter what it cost. Unmarried and never successful in romance ("Men find me threatening"), she nevertheless counted on a wide circle of friends for social and emotional support. Once a week she would manage to go to her posh gym and do an intensive aerobic workout, followed by a quick once-through on the stationary weight-resistance machines.

Avoid coffee, which can have a yo-yo mood effect. A better beverage choice is decaffeinated tea with lemon and honey.

"Listen. I have a conference call with a studio head in ninety minutes. I just need a pill that will keep the weight off. Can you write me a prescription?" asked Ms. Jones. Typical of Spirit Pathway types, Ms. Jones was trying to take control of a situation involving others while at the same time being out of control regarding herself and her cravings. As our conversation continued, it was obvious that her problem was not entirely weight. A clinical and lab evaluation indicated that her fat-to-muscle ratio was high and her bone density low. She also found herself for the first time lacking energy. These are all indicators of an advanced aging track. She was a little depressed, due in no small part to the fact that her last few sexual relationships were disastrous. "I wasn't looking for a commitment, just a little pleasure. I didn't even get that," she said. "I feel as if I'm losing control on all fronts."

Her family history revealed that part of her weight problem was genetic. Her answers to the Energy Factor questionnaire reinforced the conclusion that she was among the 25 percent or more of Americans who naturally have an abnormal glucose metabolism.

With moderately high insulin resistance, her body metabolized glucose (the body's fuel) inefficiently and allowed too much of it to be stored as fat.

Her medical history revealed the use of diet pills (amphetamines) and water pills (hydrocholorothiazide types) because of premenstrual bloating. This medication worsened her abnormal glucose metabolism by signaling her pancreas to produce more insulin. Her liver and muscle cells, however, were insensitive to receiving insulin because of her increased amount of body fat, so the excess insulin stayed in her bloodstream. Untreated, she was at high risk for adult-onset diabetes.

What she perceived as a problem with "bingeing" was actually a larger control problem caused by a dysfunction in her serotonin system. Exacerbating the problem was that she was already in a perimenopausal stage—not there yet but beginning to experience her first hot flashes, mood swings, decreased energy, and lack of vaginal lubrication. Her biomarkers confirmed that she was on an accelerated path of aging. Always the life of the party, Ms. Jones didn't even feel like going to the party anymore.

Following the recommended regimen for Spirit Pathway types, she began taking a daily supplement cocktail consisting of 50 to 200 milligrams of 5-HTP to boost her serotonin effect, 10 milligrams of DHEA in the morning to address her sluggish metabolism and replace her diminished supply of male hormones, and a nighttime dose taken intermittently as needed of melatonin to reset her sleeping pattern to a youthful state. To boost her her muscle mass and decrease her fat tissue, she began taking 2–3 grams of creatine monohydrate on an empty stomach before exercising and 3–5 grams of L-glutamine after exercise and again before sleep, also on an empty stomach.

I took her off the water pills, which were increasing her natural proclivity for insulin resistance. At night she took an extra 50 milligrams of 5-HTP when she felt out of control, and the need to binge with comfort foods. After she had been in the program sixty days, I switched her between-meals dose to 250 to 500 milligrams of L-tryptophan, to eliminate binge eating and whenever she felt agitated or anxious. At night, the critical time for Ms. Jones, I boosted her L-tryptophan dose to 2 to 3 grams to facilitate calmness and sleep.

An analysis of her food intake revealed she ate too much carbo-hydrate in the wrong way and at the wrong time. Her new regimen included a hearty breakfast with lots of lean protein to energize her for the day ahead. At lunch she ate a meal balanced between pro-tein and carbohydrates. Starchy foods such as pastas and breads dominated her dinner, which prepared her system for a peaceful night's sleep. To enhance her serotonin production she separated her simple carbohydrate intake from proteins and fats by about 90 minutes whenever possible. When food cravings hit her, she snacked on starchy foods in low-calorie amounts, such as plain French bread, puffed mini rice cakes, or dry cornflakes.

To further assist her slow metabolism, Ms. Jones began eating five small meals a day or three meals and two regular snacks. The frequent meals allowed her metabolism to stabilize, avoiding the peaks and valleys she experienced when she saved most of her caloric intake for a big dinner. She also reduced her coffee con-sumption to two cups a day and switched from one or two cocktails before dinner to a glass of red wine during her meal.

She began a moderate exercise program, beginning with 60- to 90-minute walks three times a week and a weekend class of yoga. Throughout the week she pursued "informal activity," standing when she could sit, taking stairs instead of an elevator, and so on. "My secretary thought I was crazy the first time I conference-called standing up. I told her it was the latest in biothermodynamics—all the rage in Aspen," quipped Ms. Jones.

Ninety days after she began the regimen, Ms. Jones reported that she had taken back control of her life. With her serotonin in proper balance, she is now sleeping well for the first time in five years. She wakes up refreshed. Her compulsive habits—binge eat-ing, loss of temper—are well on their way to disappearing. She was more relaxed and happier, due in small part, no doubt, to the fact that she had lost twenty pounds. She doesn't always stick to her ex-ercise regimen but makes a point of moving instead of being seden-tary whenever she can. Her love life? "Some men still think I'm controlling, but that's their problem. I can deal with it now."

Customizing Your Antiaging Regimen

~ 11 ~

Your Energy Factor

If the human body is a sophisticated biological machine, then the brain is the command center and the neurotransmitters are its communication signals. The energy needed to run the machine comes from the burning of fuel. The central source of fuel for the body comes from glucose. How and when we burn fuel defines our energy system or energy metabolism. Every cell in the body is dependent on an energy source. The brain's main fuel source is glucose, and it cannot survive long without it. The other tissues have a greater ability to oxidize (burn) other fuel sources for energy, including fats and some amino acids (the building blocks of our proteins).

When your body is working at its peak, carbohydrates, after being digested, are turned into glucose. Excess glucose can be converted into a substance called glycogen (the storage form of glucose). Glycogen is stored in muscle tissue and in the liver, ready for use as energy whenever the body needs it. If the glycogen storerooms are full, the rest of the unused ingested carbohydrates, now in the form of blood sugar, is either burned off by the body (which is why the human body exudes heat) or is stored as fat.

What happens to the protein and the fat you consume? Proteins are broken down into amino acids, which are used to form muscle and other tissue. Fat is digested, processed, and stored as, well, fat, which in itself is not a bad thing. The body calls upon its fat reserves for fuel when its glycogen storerooms become depleted.

So far so good. But like all things concerned with the human body, the system begins to break down with age. For most of us, the decline starts around the age of thirty-five. Insulin begins to lose its "glucose disposal capacity"—its ability to move glucose into cells to fuel the body and to promote protein synthesis. To compensate, the pancreas produces more insulin. But tissues lose their receptivity to insulin with aging and with conditions such as obesity, genetic predisposition, and certain drugs. As a result, the body becomes *insulin resistant.*

Insulin serves as a shuttle for getting glucose into the cells and turning on protein synthesis. Insulin resistance is the condition in which the cells become less receptive to insulin, requiring more of it to do its job. This in turn produces excessive amounts of insulin in the bloodstream, which ultimately has a toxic effect on the body. And therein lies the dual nature of insulin: not enough, and the body can't make its primary energy source; too much, and it becomes very pro-aging. The excess insulin in the blood contributes to a wide range of conditions associated with aging, including increased free radicals, oxidation damage to cells, non-insulin-dependent diabetes, obesity, abnormal lipid levels, heart disease, strokes, high blood pressure, brain inflammation, and brain aging.

To make matters worse, we have accelerated the demise of our own energy metabolic systems. It is estimated that since 1935 the incidence of diabetes has increased 750 percent, just about the same increase as our sugar consumption. What's the connection? Not all carbohydrates are created equal, at least not in producing an insulin response. Carbohydrates can be categorized into two basic groups: low glycemic; the slowly digested, resistant starches; and high glycemic, which are quickly digested and absorbed. Low-glycemic, high fiber carbohydrate foods, such as plums and lentils, are digested and enter the bloodstream slowly, producing a slower, lower insulin response. The high-glycemic starches, such as puffed rice cakes and French bread, are rapidly broken down and enter the bloodstream quickly, provoking a large and rapid insulin surge.

Perhaps a better way to think of the two types of carbohydrates is natural (unrefined) and manufactured (refined). When the cell walls of a grain are removed or broken down (as with white bread or instant rice), the carbohydrate becomes more easily digested and absorbed. Not too long ago—the late fifteenth century, to be precise—there were virtually no refined carbohydrates in the average person's diet. There was no such thing as white bread, instant rice, sugar-coated cereals, and snack cakes. Sugars were available in the forms of honey and maple syrup, but they were used sparingly as sweetening agents and not as a daily staple. The carbohydrates people consumed in the old days contained more natural fiber.

The human body can accommodate vast differences in dietary habits; one only has to contrast Japanese and Mexican cuisine to be convinced. However, the body's metabolism is designed to break down the carbohydrates and remove sugars from high-fiber foods. Foods with natural fibers have cell walls that are more intact than refined foods. It takes more time for the digestive juices to fight through and attack the starch-sugar chains, thus releasing simple sugars into the bloodstream. Since this process takes more time, a simple sugar like glucose is "pulsed" into the body rather than "jolted" in by the rapid breakdown and assimilation.

By eating a constant diet high in refined and easily digested carbohydrates, such as cornflakes, cooked carrots, brown rice, white rice, sweet corn, raisins, crackers, pastry, and cookies, your insulin levels will keep climbing and make you fat. Chronic ingestion of these foods leads to abnormal glucose metabolism (AGM), and can lead to insulin resistance. The aging process accelerates rapidly when your blood glucose and insulin levels remain high. The eyes, nerves, and kidneys are the first to suffer, being more sensitive than other tissue to sugar overload.

What is more, when we eat lots of refined sugar, what isn't burned off is stored as fat. With our sugar consumption rising 750 percent over the last sixty years or so, it's obvious why America has become the land of the fat.

America: Land of the Fat

How fat are we as a nation? About 58 million Americans are clinically obese, defined as 20 percent heavier than their ideal weight. About 50 percent of all women and 25 percent of all men are overweight, according to survey studies. The danger of rail-thin fashion models being served up by the mass media as models of health

Figure 2

Body Mass Index (BMI)*

BMI	25	26	27	28	29	30	31	32	33	34	35	36	37	38	39	40	41	42	43	44	45	46	47	48	49	50
HEIGHT			At risk ▶ WEIGHT (In Pounds)																							
4'10"	119	124	129	134	138	143	148	153	158	162	167	172	177	181	186	191	194	199	203	208	213	218	222	227	232	237
4'11"	124	128	133	138	143	148	153	158	163	168	173	178	183	188	193	198	201	206	211	215	220	224	230	235	240	245
5'	128	133	138	143	148	153	158	164	169	174	179	184	189	194	199	204	207	213	218	223	228	233	238	243	248	253
5'1"	132	137	143	148	153	158	164	169	174	180	185	190	195	201	206	211	214	220	225	230	235	241	246	251	257	262
5'2"	136	142	147	153	158	164	169	175	180	186	191	196	202	207	213	218	221	227	232	238	243	249	254	260	265	271
5'3"	141	146	152	158	163	169	175	180	186	192	197	203	208	214	220	225	229	234	240	246	251	257	262	268	274	279
5'4"	145	151	157	163	169	174	180	186	192	198	203	209	215	221	227	233	236	242	248	253	259	265	271	277	282	288
5'5"	150	156	162	168	174	180	186	192	198	204	210	216	222	228	234	240	243	249	255	261	267	273	279	285	291	297
5'6"	155	161	167	173	179	185	192	198	204	210	216	223	229	235	241	247	251	257	263	269	276	282	290	294	300	307
5'7"	159	166	172	178	185	191	198	204	210	217	223	229	236	242	248	255	260	266	271	277	284	290	297	303	309	316
5'8"	164	171	177	184	190	197	203	210	217	223	230	236	243	249	256	263	266	272	279	286	293	299	306	312	319	325
5'9"	169	176	182	189	196	203	209	216	223	230	237	243	250	257	264	270	274	281	288	294	301	308	315	321	328	335
5'10"	174	181	188	195	202	209	216	223	230	236	243	250	257	264	271	278	282	289	296	303	310	317	324	331	338	345
5'11"	179	186	193	200	207	215	222	229	236	243	250	258	265	272	279	286	290	297	305	313	319	326	333	340	348	355
6'	184	191	199	206	213	221	228	235	243	250	258	265	272	280	287	294	298	306	313	321	328	335	343	350	357	365
6'1"	189	197	204	212	219	227	234	242	250	257	265	272	280	287	295	303	307	313	322	328	337	345	352	360	367	375
6'2"	194	202	210	218	225	233	241	249	256	264	272	280	288	295	303	311	315	323	331	339	346	354	362	370	378	385
6'3"	200	208	216	224	232	240	247	255	263	271	279	287	295	303	311	319	324	332	340	348	356	364	372	380	388	396
6'4"	205	213	221	230	238	246	254	262	271	279	287	295	303	312	320	328	332	341	349	357	365	373	382	390	398	406

* BMI is calculated by dividing weight (in kilograms) by height[2] (in meters[2]).

notwithstanding, fat is more than an issue of being attractive. Each year, 300,000 patients die from obesity-related complications—a figure exceeded only by smoking as the leading cause of preventable death in the United States.

Fat promotes aging in several ways. Lugging around excess weight grinds down the body's biomechanical system, making joints deteriorate more quickly, in turn restricting movement and

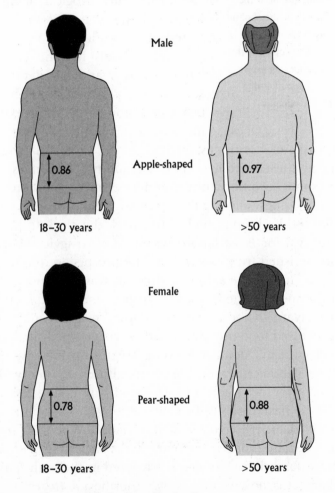

Figure 3—"Gut Versus Butt Fat Distribution"
With age, men typically gain weight in their abdomen, producing an apple shaped fat distribution. On the other hand, women tend to gain weight around their buttocks and thighs, resulting in a pear shape. The indexes ranging from .78 to .97 are waist-to-hip ratios; a smaller number indicates a greater hip-to-waist fat distribution, while a higher number indicates the waist is closer to the size of the hips.

making exercise more difficult, which begins a downward spiral to a sedentary, pro-aging lifestyle. Overweight people don't live very long. Have you seen many obese people who are seventy-five years or older?

Never eat sweets, especially foods containing refined sugars or honey, before bedtime unless you are low in serotonin and need the relaxation effect. The body's metabolism of refined sugar produces insulin very quickly. In turn, insulin suppresses the release of the super-antiaging growth hormone, which is released during the first ninety minutes of sleep.

The underlying causes of excessive fat in the body also encourages the production of free radicals. Obesity starts a whole cascade of abnormal physiological aging events, with just about every system of the body affected. The cardiovascular system suffers; blood vessels become clogged and inflamed rapidly, and blood pressure increases, adversely affecting the brain, kidneys, heart, and blood flow to the extremities. Obesity inhibits the immune system and depresses levels of hormones, including the very antiaging growth hormone and testosterone in men. The joints at the knees, hips, ankles, and spine become arthritic, and it becomes painful to move.

When it comes to losing that excess weight, Nature has played a cruel joke on the human body. Turn back the clock to the Ice Age when survival for *homo sapiens* was a daily struggle. Many of our ancestors perished from starvation. The prospect of too much food didn't exist. In fact, the ability to store fat was an important advantage for the species. The fittest were those who stored fat the best.

Fast-forward to the twentieth century when readily available, highly processed food products (loaded with refined sugars and fat) combined with a sedentary lifestyle creates an increasingly overweight population, at least in Western cultures. In theory, the average person should be able to lose weight by eating less. But the human body hasn't evolved quickly enough to accommodate the excesses of twentieth-century dietary habits. When we try to lose weight, especially quickly, the body harks back to its Ice Age mode and thinks starvation. A switch is triggered in the brain's hypothalamus that turns down your body's thermostat (to conserve heat and energy), which sends the body into a fat-and-calorie-preserving mode. Now when you eat, almost everything is turned to fat, and you're worse off than when you started dieting.

Insulin Resistance and Metabolic Syndrome X

All things not being equal, each of us is born with a genetic hand of cards, a combination of good and bad that affects everything from looks to personality. The same is true with each individual's ability to respond to sugars. That's why Joe can stuff his face with all the carbohydrates he wants and not gain a pound, while Jim, try as he might, gains weight even when he's trying his best to eat heathfully.

Studies show that about one in four of us has a predisposition toward being "insulin resistant." That means the insulin doesn't work as efficiently as it should, that is, it takes more insulin than normal to get the normal physiological result of transporting glucose into the cell. Scientists call this condition *abnormal glucose metabolism* (AGM). The end result is usually excess weight and an accelerated aging track.

Get in the habit of reading labels. By federal law, all packaged or processed food must contain a label listing its caloric content and its percentage of carbohydrates, proteins, fats, and its sugar and sodium content.

Among the 25 percent who are genetically inclined to AGM, there are degrees of insulin resistance. Nutritional researcher Jeffrey Bland, Ph.D., has identified three levels of insulin resistance: (1) normal, (2) mild to moderate, and (3) significant. The third level is also known as Metabolic Syndrome X, a term coined by another researcher, Gerald M. Reaven, M.D., in the 1980s. Many Metabolic Syndrome X sufferers are fat because they have seriously abnormal glucose metabolism (severe AGM).

Metabolic Syndrome X patients typically have an apple-shaped body, with fat distributed around and in the gut. There is an increased waist-to-hip ratio (the circumference of the waist is much greater than it should be in relation to the hip circumference). With age, women natually put on weight in their thighs and hips, developing a pear shape, so an apple shape on women could be an indicator of Metabolic Syndrome X. For men, who typically gain weight in their upper bodies with age, the signs of Metabolic Syndrome X can be more subtle, although a huge belly that hangs over the belt line is a good indicator. While Metabolic Syndrome X is associated with excess weight, being fat is not an absolute requisite. In his study, Reaven estimated that 25 percent of Metabolic Syndrome X sufferers were not obese.

Precautions

The questionnaire below is designed to indicate where you fall on the glucose metabolism spectrum. Your score will direct you to one of four energy regimens, the second most important factor (after your Mind, Body, Spirit Pathway) in developing your Personal Antiaging Regimen.

As always, precautions must be taken if you are currently under treatment or using medication, especially for hypo- or hyper-glycemia, hypertension, atherosclerosis, or endocrinological disorders. Consult with your doctor if you have a preexisting condition or a family history of these diseases. If you haven't had a glucose tolerance test recently, have one taken with insulin levels measured along with glucose levels. The two most important values are the fasting glucose/insulin levels and the two-hour glucose/insulin levels, if you are doing the short two-hour screening test and not the five-hour study. Your doctor may want you to do the five-hour test if the two-hour test results look suspicious. This may be a good time to get a glucose/carbohydrate challenge test from your doctor as you embark on your antiaging regimen.

If you are an insulin-dependent diabetic or have been diagnosed as having adult-onset diabetes, then skip this questionnaire and consult with your physician regarding your diet and medications.

ENERGY METABOLISM QUOTIENT

Answer every question "yes" or "no" to the best of your ability. If the answer to a question is yes, write the corresponding points in the blank at the beginning of each question. Score 0 if the answer is no.

____ 1. Measure your blood pressure. If your blood pressure is elevated, score 4 points.

Note: You no longer need a doctor to measure your blood pressure. Most drugstores and even malls have vending-type machines that accurately measure your blood pressure.

____ 2. Are you on medicine that treats your elevated blood pressure? If yes, score 8 points.

____ 3. Measure the circumference of your waist at the level of the belly button after breathing out and relaxing. Then measure your hip circumference at the broadest area where the hip-bones stick out. Divide the waist size by the hip size.

If the number (waist-to-hip ratio) is between .90 and .95, score 4 points.

If the ratio is .96 to 1.0, score 8 points.

If the number is greater than 1.0, score 12 points.

___ 4. What is your body-mass index? Find your BMI index by cross-referencing your height and weight on the chart on page 142.

Under 25, score 0 points

25, score 4 points

26, score 8 points

27, score 10 points

28, score 12 points

30 or over, score 15 points

___ 5. Do this simple home blood sugar test. Buy a glucose instrument, a glucometer, at your local drugstore. The cost is from $50 to $80.

A. Eat a diet of 150 to 200 grams of carbohydrates daily for three days before the test, especially if you have been on a carbohydrate-restricted diet. Fast overnight, having no food and drinking only water for 10 to 12 hours.

B. The morning after the 10- to 12-hour fast, prick your finger to get a drop of blood and measure it with the glucometer.

If your fasting blood sugar is 110–115, score 5 points.

If 115–135, score 10 points.

If 135–155, score 20 points.

If 155–175, score 30 points.

If greater than 175, score 40 points.

C. Eat your normal breakfast or have a Glucola drink (available at drugstores) containing 75 grams of glucose.

D. Wait two hours and measure the blood glucose level again:

If it is 140–160, score 20 points.

If it is 160–180, score 30 points.

If it is more than 180, score 40 points.

___ 6. Do you have any blood relatives with diabetes who take insulin injections? If yes, score 10 points.

___ 7. Do you have blood relatives who are diabetic and are being treated with oral medications? If yes, score 8 points.

____ 8. Do you have blood relatives who have been diagnosed as diabetic but are treated with diet and exercise alone? If yes, score 6 points.

____ 9. Do you constantly crave carbohydrates, such as sweets, breads, and pastas, and then after eating them feel weak or faint? If yes, score 4 points.

____ 10. Have you ever been on a self-imposed diet where you lost and gained over 20 pounds? If yes, score 12 points.

____ 11. Have you ever been on a medically prescribed diet for obesity? If yes, score 20 points.

____ 12. Based on your last physical examination, do you have elevated cholesterol levels or other bad fats in your blood high enough so that your doctor indicated you might require medicine if they did not go down with exercise, diet, and lifestyle changes? (If you haven't had a physical exam in the last year, this is a good time to get one.) If yes, score 10 points.

____ 13. Do you use water pills or a diuretic such as the hydrochlorothiazide type (Dyazide, Diuril, HydroDIURIL, and so forth) to lower your blood pressure? If yes, score 15 points.

____ 14. Do you use female hormones, such as estrogen? If yes, score 8 points.

____ 15. Do you continually use the cortisone type of medicine, such as prednisone? If yes, score 20 points.

____ 16. Have you had more than 3 cortisone injections in the past 6 months? If yes, score 10 points.

____ 17. Are you using beta-blocker medication, such as the propranolol type (Inderal, Levatol, Tenormin, Lopressor, and others)? If yes, score 15 points.

____ 18. Do you drink coffee or other caffeinated beverages, such as cola, or use caffeine supplements more than once a day? If yes, score 4 points.

____ 19. If you are a woman, have you ever been diagnosed as having polycysytic ovary syndrome? If yes, score 25 points.

____ 20. Have you ever been diagnosed as having any diseases of the blood vessels of the heart or elsewhere? If yes, score 15 points.

____ 21. Have you ever been diagnosed as producing too much cortisol from your adrenal glands and having high blood cortisol levels? If yes, score 20 points.

INTERPRETING YOUR SCORE

Tally your score and find your energy-glucose metabolism category below.

Total Score

0–50   Normal: You are one of the lucky ones. Your glucose-metabolic system is working efficiently. But keep in mind that after thirty-five, your glucose metabolism will begin to deteriorate, and you can expect to gain weight—especially between ages forty and sixty. To lose those extra pounds, restrict your diet to no more than 2,000 calories a day if you're a man of normal BMI and not exceedingly active physically; 1,500 calories a day if you're a woman with average-normal BMI and not exceedingly active physically.

Avoid low-fiber processed foods that are quickly digested and absorbed into your bloodstream, that is, high-glycemic types such as crackers, bagels, puffed rice cakes, and cornflakes. (See page 261 for the Glycemic Index of common foods.) Too many high-glycemic foods can lead to the promotion of free radicals, inflammation, and accelerated aging.

51–150   Mild—Level 1 Abnormal Glucose Metabolism (AGM-1): You probably have a slight degree of abnormal glucose metabolism with elevated insulin levels and a decreased capacity for "glucose disposal" from the bloodstream. That means your cells are somewhat insensitive to the action of insulin. The glucose is not being efficiently removed from the bloodstream and put into the cells where it belongs. The end result is that there is excess blood sugar with nowhere to go. This starts a toxic cascade, which can produce a measurable amount of excessive oxidative stress on the whole body.

At this level of AGM and insulin insensitivity, your goals should be to reduce excess body fat and improve your body composition by a better diet and low-intensity moderate exercise. By decreasing body fat, your cells become alive and soak up the blood sugar as they are supposed to. When you lose fat mass and build muscle mass, your body automatically increases its metabolic rate. You burn an increased number of calories even when you are not even exercising.

Here are specific recommendations for Level 1:

Diet:

Meals should consist of 60 percent unrefined, low-glycemic, high-fiber carbohydrates, 20 percent proteins, and 20 percent fat/oils. Don't eat carbohydrates alone, as a rule, unless it is a low-glycemic vegetable or fruit snack. (See chapter 17 for the index to low glycemic carbohydrate foods.) Eat at least three servings weekly of foods rich in omega-3 oils (such as dark-meat fish).

Supplements:

Make the following modifications to the supplements recommended in the Antiaging Cocktail and your Mind-Body-Spirit Pathway regimen. Do not exceed the maximum safe dosages. (See chapter 15, page 217, for a guide to maximum dosages.)

ANTIOXIDANT GROUP
Increase vitamin E to 600 IU daily
Increase CoQ10 to 100 mg daily
Increase zinc (chelate) to 20–30 mg daily
Increase selenium (chelate, aspartate) to 200 mcg daily
Increase N-acetyl L-cysteine to 600 mg, daily
Increase vitamin C to 1,000 mg daily

MITOCHONDRIAL PROTECTORS
Increase acetyl L-carnitine to 250 mg daily
Increase alpha lipoic acid to 250 mg daily

B VITAMIN GROUP
Increase B_3 (niacinamide) to 200 mg twice a day
Increase folic acid to 400 mg twice a day

MACROMINERAL
Increase magnesium to 400 mg, daily

TRACE MINERAL GROUP
Add 500 mcg daily of vanadyl sulfate
Adjust chromium to 100 mcg, twice a day with food

MISCELLANEOUS
Increase inositol to 1,000 mg daily
Increase biotin to 200 mcg daily

Add L-carnitine: 500 mg daily
Increase betaine HCL (trimethyl glycine HCL) to 400 mg daily

HERBS AND SPICES
Increase garlic to 2 cloves three times a day or 2 capsules 3 times a day with food

SMART OILS
Switch to omega-3 fish oil, consisting of 300 mg EPA and 200 mg of DHA per gram: $^1/_2$ teaspoon or 2–3 grams daily

NEW SUPPLEMENT FOR AGM-1
DHEA, 5 mg in the morning
Men can increase the micronized DHEA dose from 5 milligrams to 20 milligrams. Studies have shown that DHEA can have an insulin-lowering effect. Above this level, the sex hormones (free serum or salivary testosterone and the total serum estrogens), glucose, PSA, and insulin levels need to be monitored by your physician. Women can increase micronized DHEA to 15 milligrams. Above this level your doctor should be consulted. Using high doses of DHEA can potentially contribute to liver cancer, prostate cancer in men, breast cancer in women, and can disturb your hormonal balance. Low doses must be used until long-term human studies are completed.

Exercise:
30 minutes of an aerobic exercise 3 times a week, such as fast walking, jogging, or bicycling, and 20–30 minutes of weight training twice a week

Stress Management:
By decreasing stress, you can decrease your cortisol levels, bring your energy-glucose metabolism toward a normal state, and increase your DHEA levels. This all helps to keep your blood sugar level and insulin in better balance. For more advice on stress management, see chapter 13.

151–250 Moderate—Level 2 Moderately Abnormal Glucose Metabolism (AGM-2) with Insulin Resistance: Chances are you are overweight, perhaps even clinically obese. Your blood levels show some increase in insulin and increased levels of triglycerides and an increase of the low-density type of lipids called LDL. The blood sugars run in the high-normal range.

More intense and increased frequency of exercise and dietary intervention are needed to help reverse your abnormal Level 2 Glucose Metabolism (AGM-2). Stress may be exacerbating your poor metabolism by increasing cortisol output that elevates your already high glucose and insulin levels. Follow this advice in conjunction with your Mind-Body-Spirit Pathway regimen:

Diet:
Food intake should consist of 50 percent unrefined low-glycemic high-fiber carbohydrates, 25 percent protein, and 25 percent fats/oils. There should be less than 10 percent fat from saturated fats/oils such as meats, lard, or the tropical oils. Consume at least 3 servings weekly of omega-3 oil-rich foods, such as cold-water fish or dark-meat fish, or the equivalent in supplements.

Add soluble fiber from oat bran, apple pectin, cellulose gum, and so forth, or try a fiber-loaded formula with both soluble and insoluble fiber. The formula should be taken alone between meals, mixed in water or a diluted, unsweetened juice. Do not take supplements with the formula since it may bind them, preventing them from getting absorbed. Try to get a total fiber intake of 25–30 grams per day.

Supplements:
Make the following modifications to the supplements recommended in the Antiaging Cocktail and your Mind-Body-Spirit Pathway regimen. Don't exceed the maximum safe dosages.

ANTIOXIDANT GROUP
Increase vitamin E to 800 IU
Increase vitamin C to 1 gram, four times daily.
Increase CoQ10 to 150 mg daily
Increase N-acetyl L-cysteine to 600 mg twice daily

MITOCHONDRIAL PROTECTORS
Increase acetyl L-carnitine to 500 mg daily
Increase alpha lipoic acid to 500 mg daily

B VITAMIN GROUP

Increase B_3 (niacinamide) to 200 mg three times a day

Increase B_{12} to 500 mcg twice daily

Increase folic acid to 800 mg twice daily

MACROMINERALS

Increase magnesium to 600 mg daily

TRACE MINERAL GROUP

Add vanadyl sulfate: 500–1,000 mcg daily

Adjust chromium to 200 mcg twice daily

MISCELLANEOUS

Increase inositol to 2,000 mg daily

Increase biotin to 200 mcg daily

Add L-carnitine: 500 mg twice daily

Increase betaine HCL (trimethyl glycine HCL) to 800 mg daily

HERBS AND SPICES

Increase garlic to 2 cloves three times a day or 2 capsules 3 times a day with food

SMART OILS

Switch to omega-3 fish oil, consisting of 300 mg EPA and 200 mg of DHA per gram: $^1/_2$ teaspoon or 2–3 grams twice daily.

NEW SUPPLEMENT FOR AGM-2

DHEA, 5–10 mg in the morning

Exercise:

To decrease your fat mass and increase your lean mass, your exercise regimen should consist of low-intensity, fat-burning exercises from 60 minutes to 90 minutes, four to five times per week. Alternate walking with bike riding (treadmills and stationary bikes are fine). Weight-bearing exercises are preferable to swimming. Alternate aerobic exercise with a weight-training exercise program of 20–30 minutes twice a week. Weight training can stimulate muscle growth in the upper body and elsewhere. See chapter 9 for more information on beginning a weight-training program.

Stress Management:
To decrease stress/cortisol levels, start a daily practice of 15–20 minutes of quiet time per day consisting of meditation and other mind/body-quieting activity. Choose from yoga, tai chi, and other mind/body-balancing exercises.

251 or more   Metabolic Syndrome X—Level 3 Extremely Abnormal Glucose Metabolism (AGM-3) with Severe Insulin Resistance: Your test score indicates that you may be suffering from Metabolic Syndrome X, a severe imbalance of your glucose metabolism with insulin insensitivity and elevated blood glucose. This is a condition with potentially serious health effects, and consultation with a knowledgeable health professional is strongly advised. The following can be included in your restorative regimen:

Diet:
Eat frequent smaller balanced meals, at least six a day, instead of three large meals to help reduce and moderate insulin response. All meals should consist of 50 percent unrefined carbohydrates, 30 percent protein, and 20 percent fats/oils. Make sure you eat low-glycemic carbohydrates containing a lot of fiber. Raw foods provoke less of an insulin response than cooked foods. Baked carbohydrate foods stimulate insulin less than boiled ones. See chapter 17 for dietary choices.

Also, eat three servings or more per week of fish rich in omega-3 oil (cold-water fish or dark-meat fish). Take 2 daily servings of a high-fiber supplement formula preferably soluble up to 10–15 grams, daily. Do *not* take other supplements with your fiber formula since it may bind them and prevent them from getting absorbed.

For between-meal snacks, mix a soy protein isolate or a non-soy vegetable protein (for soy-allergic people) with water, a low-calorie juice drink, nonfat soy milk, or some other beverage that is low calorie but *not* fruit juice! Along with the protein drinks have a small handful of dry-roasted, unsalted peanuts, almonds, or sunflower seeds. With nuts, these drinks can take the place of some of your meals. For the average man on a 2,000-calorie diet, he needs to eat 330 calories six times per day. A woman on a 1,500-calorie program needs 250 calories six times a day.

Supplements:
Your system is generating a lot of free radicals, and you are far out of balance in many systems, which necessitates medical supervision. To reverse the effects of oxidative stress and free-radical damage, begin a supplement program of intensive mitochondrial support and an antioxidant boosting program combined with a low-calorie diet of raw fruits and vegetables full of phytonutrients and antioxidants.

Make the following modifications to the supplements recommended in the Antiaging Cocktail and your Pathway regimen. Do not exceed the maximum safe dosages. (See pp. 289–291 for a guide to maximum dosages.)

ANTIOXIDANT GROUP
Increase the natural mixed carotenes to 20 mg daily
Increase vitamin E to 1,000 IU as long as you have no known
    bleeding problems or are not taking anticoagulant medications
Increase vitamin C to 6 grams daily, divided into 3 doses
Increase CoQ10 to 200 mg daily
Increase N-acetyl L-cysteine to 600 mg three times a day
Increase selenium to 300 mcg daily

MITOCHONDRIAL PROTECTORS
Increase acetyl L-carnitine to 1 to 1^1/$_2$ grams daily in the morning
Increase alpha lipoic acid to 500–750 mg daily

B VITAMIN GROUP
Increase B$_3$ (niacinamide) to 400 mg three times a day
Increase B$_{12}$ to 500 mcg twice daily
Increase folic acid to 2,000 mcg twice daily

MACROMINERALS
Increase magnesium to 600–800 mg daily

TRACE MINERAL GROUP
Add vanadyl sulfate: 2–5 mg daily
Adjust chromium to 300 mcg twice daily

MISCELLANEOUS
Increase inositol to 3,000 mg daily
Increase biotin to 300 mcg daily
Add L-carnitine: 1 gram twice daily
Increase betaine HCL (trimethyl glycine HCL) to 1,000 mg daily

HERBS AND SPICES
Increase garlic to 2 cloves three times a day or two capsules 3 times a day with food.

SMART OILS
Switch to omega-3 fish oil, consisting of 300 mg EPA and 200 mg of DHA per gram: ³/₄ teaspoon or 4 grams twice daily

Always take your antioxidants (especially the vitamin E fat-soluble group, CoQ10 and alpha lipoic acid) *before* the oils or with them to decrease the oil oxidation potential and free-radical formation.

NEW SUPPLEMENT FOR AGM-3
DHEA, 10 mg in the morning

Medications:
Meridia (scientific name: sibuturamine hydrochloride) is the latest Next Big Thing in the weight-loss industry. Released in February 1998, the pill has already become the most successful weight-control supplement ever marketed, but I am not sold on it yet. The pill suppresses appetite by enhancing the body's serotonin effect. That in itself is nothing novel, and, in my own clinical experience, has not proven effective. It is also not appropriate for anyone with high blood pressure.

Another new weight-loss drug, currently awaiting FDA approval, is Xenocal (active ingredient: orlistat xenocal). It works by blocking the body's absorption of fat in food, which it does, but, in the process, it also blocks those fats that are good for you as well as fat-soluble vitamins. Reported side effects include diarrhea, and it may be associated with an increased risk of cancer.

Both drugs approach the problem of obesity from a one-size-fits-all perspective, but in fact, weight control demands a multidimensional solution. The day may yet come when a single pill can cure obesity. In the meantime, a personalized program that integrates supplements, diet and nutrition, and exercise is required.

Exercise:

If you're a classic Metabolism Syndrome X sufferer, it's likely you are clinically obese. These individuals are at higher risk for cardiovascular complications. Exercise must be done in a much milder and less intense way than in the two previously discussed AGM levels. The body is in a highly stressed, oxidative state so that intense aerobics would only make things worse. Any exercise program must proceed slowly and in consultation with a physician and, optimally, a physical trainer.

A typical beginner's weekly exercise program would include:

◆ Low-intensity stationary bike riding or treadmill or easy outdoor walking. Break into a sweat and then keep your heart rate at 55–60 percent of the maximum for your age.

◆ Gentle stretching and easy weight training. The idea at this level is not to do exhaustive exercise. Do not get too winded. When your weight and blood pressure are improved, you can then increase the intensity.

◆ Mind/body exercise such as tai chi, Qi gong (an ancient Chinese breathing and movement exercise), yoga, and meditation are highly encouraged for this very stress-loaded condition. Find some mind/body activity that makes you feel greater harmony and more at peace within yourself and with the world.

~ 12 ~

Your Sex Factor

Any serious antiaging regimen must figure the role of the sex hormones into the formula. The female hormone system, which consists of the estrogen family (estrone, estrogen, and estriol) and progesterone, and the male hormone system (testosterone and dihydrotestosterone) are integrally linked to the aging process.

Every individual has an ideal sex hormone zone. For both men and women the ideal level is a matter of balancing testosterone and estrogen to a ratio that promotes antiaging. Let me repeat that. Both men and women need adequate levels of testosterone and estrogen to maintain an effective antiaging program.

Testosterone is converted into estrogen by the aromatase enzyme in both sexes. With age the ratio of testosterone to estrogen changes for a number of reasons, and this change is accompanied by an increased percentage of body fat that affects both sexes. For men the cause is often an increase in aromatase enzyme activity. More estrogen is produced in relation to testosterone, resulting in a decline in the body's energy metabolic system.

The connection between obesity and low testosterone sometimes shows up in some middle-aged men in a condition biologists call "central adiposity" or what the layman calls "beer gut." Men who have this pattern can have a fairly normal fat distribution except around their belly. From a profile they look as if they are pregnant. Central obesity can be a sign of low testosterone, especially if the testes have become smaller in size and the person has become super-obese. In general, obese men have lower testosterone concentrations than nonobese men.

The central adiposity condition is rarer in women but more dangerous. If a woman develops central abdominal obesity, she is eight times more at risk to die from a heart attack.

Centrally obese persons in general have increased risk of heart disease, stroke, and hypertension. Estrogen replacement in postmenopausal women and testosterone replacement in men with low testosterone concentrations decrease central abdominal fat.

If you take away nothing else from this chapter, understand that both men and women need testosterone and estrogen throughout their lives. For men it is important to know that testosterone is a "prohormone," or the stuff from which two other hormones are made: the male hormone dihydrotestosterone and the female hormone known as estrogen. The overall effect of testosterone is the result of the combined effects of testosterone plus dihydrotestosterone and estrogen. When you add up all three, you have the male hormone sex factor.

Female Sex Factor

The female sex hormone factor is a little more complicated and has more players in the game: the three estrogens (estrone, estradiol, and estriol), progesterone, plus testosterone. Determining the appropriate hormone ratios and the relationships among and between these five hormones is one of the most important antiaging strategies.

Estrogen is widely used by women to diminish the effects of menopause, which can include hot flashes, night sweats, vaginal dryness, and dramatic mood swings. In fact, Premarin, an estrogen made from the urine of pregnant horses, is the number one brand-name prescription drug in the U.S. with about 44 million prescriptions written every year. Premarin is taken by between one-sixth and one-fourth of all women entering menopause or in menopause, which virtually all women experience between the ages of forty and fifty-five.

It is understandable to think of the female sex hormones as impacting only the sexual function, but in truth estrogen receptors can be found in three hundred tissues throughout the body including the brain, liver, and bones. Estrogen increases the amount of an enzyme in the brain that is necessary for the production of acetylcholine, which as we learned earlier is a neurotransmitter essential to a well-functioning memory system. This may be one of the reasons that studies indicate maintaining youthful levels of estrogen can prevent the delay or the onset of Alzheimer's disease in women by as much as two-thirds.

Estrogen can also prevent many pathological conditions associated with aging, including heart disease, osteoporosis, and colon cancer. And it helps maintain supple skin, prevents the atrophy of the female genitalia, and preserves strong teeth and bones.

But estrogen replacement therapy (ERT) is not for all women. Indeed, there is a continuing debate as to whether ERT is even "natural," that women should be allowed to age gracefully without the societal and peer pressure of being forever young or eternally feminine. That argument misses the point: In terms of evolutionary development of our human species, there is nothing natural about women living healthy lives well beyond their reproductive years. Until this century, women died shortly after their ovaries stopped producing estrogen. The estrogen decline in postmenopausal women is so severe that the average fifty-year-old man has more estrogen than his distaff counterpart. While at much smaller levels than women's, men's estrogen supplies do not decline with age, which may be the reason that twice as many women have Alzheimer's as do men.

The degree or amount of suffering a woman goes through at menopause depends on many variables: genetics, smoking, drinking, diet, exercise, lifestyle, and country of origin and culture, among others. That menopause has a cultural factor is evidenced by Japanese women, who outlive American women by six or seven years and have only 50 percent of the cases of osteoporosis even though their bones have less mass and the intake of milk is low. Japanese women also have 75 percent fewer deaths from heart disease, 60 percent to 70 percent fewer deaths from breast cancer, and substantially less ovarian cancer. In Japanese culture there is no word for "hot flash." In Japan and other Asian cultures women experience fewer symptoms and usually don't seek medical help for menopausal symptoms. How do you explain this? Traditionally, women in Japan and Asia don't drink much alcohol and don't smoke. And the traditional kind of rural Asian diets are full of phytonutrients and antioxidants with vegetable proteins, mainly from soy.

Philosophy and culture aside, there is an association between ERT and cancer in U.S. women, particularly breast cancer and, to a lesser degree, cancer of the ovaries and uterus. The risk of cancer can be mitigated by using the lowest effective dosage as possible. After a woman and her physician have decided to choose ERT, they must work together closely to determine her optimal and effective level and the possibility of combination therapy with progesterone or hormones (testosterone, DHEA, etc.). Estrogen is available by prescription only and should remain that way. If you are using synthetic sex hormones, such as Premarin, Provera, or methyl testosterone, have your doctor switch you to the natural forms of progesterone, estrogen, and natural testosterone. Research shows the natural forms of hormones are safer over the long run.

The other primary female hormone, progesterone, is frequently combined with estrogen to reduce the risk of uterine cancer. Progesterone in a weak cream form is available for sale directly to the public. Some women are starting to use natural micronized progesterone (the form less likely to be broken down by the liver), available in supplements, to treat some of the common symptoms of menopause such as hot flashes.

Women who don't want estrogen hormone replacement therapy can seek to modulate the effects of estrogen-progesterone loss during and before the perimenopausal time periods from phytonutrient dietary sources. The best source of dietary estrogen is soybeans and soybean products, including tofu, soy milk, miso, soy burgers, soy nuts, soy flour, soy protein powders, roasted soy butter, and textured vegetable protein. The soy isolate protein powders contain a lot of isoflavone phytonutrients, but we don't know yet if these isolated forms are as beneficial as those in the whole food form. In the meantime, it's best not to rely on any one particular soy-derived product and stay with the whole beans, tofu, and other unrefined forms.

Contrary to popular opinion, Mexican wild yams are not a good source for hormones. Since the Mexican wild yam is used pharmaceutically as the raw material to make sex hormones, the notion has arisen that you can just use a yam extract cream and ingest wild Mexican yam products to get progesterone or some other hormonal effect. This is not a reliable or cost-effective method for treating perimenopausal symptoms or the diseases associated with menopause.

There are a number of vitamins and herbal and botanical remedies for perimenopausal and menopausal symptoms, including bioflavonoids (the inner white peel of citrus fruits); black cohosh, which has an estrogenic effect and may not be good for women at risk for breast cancer; garden sage; vitamin E; dong quai (a naturally occurring phytoestrogen); licorice root; and red raspberry. [See chapter 16 for more information on these substances.] Cabbage contains a phytonutrient, indole-3-carbinol, that according to one research study reduced significantly the level of a type of estrogen known to promote breast cancer.

While estrogen and progesterone are the primary female sex hormones, women also make a small degree of testosterone—small but very important. For both men *and* women, testosterone affects the sex drive and sets the mind, mood, and fantasies for having sex. A testosterone deficiency can leave some women feeling sexually listless, depressed, and uninterested. Women also need a small level of testosterone to keep their muscles and bones strong. Women who use estrogen replacement generally have lower concentrations of testosterone. Replacement therapy with testosterone seems to work best in those women who had a very low level to start with. Most women get a big boost from very little testosterone since they naturally begin with low levels.

Do you have a need for sex hormone replacement therapy? Is it worth the risk? Ultimately, this must be decided by you in consultation with your physician, but the following questionnaire will help you determine the answers to these questions.

FEMALE SEX FACTOR QUESTIONNAIRE

_____ 1. Are you having memory lapses that are becoming disturbing to you? If yes, score 2 points.

_____ 2. Do you have a family history of Alzheimer's disease? If yes, score 3 points.

_____ 3. Do you experience hot flashes almost hourly? If yes, score 3 points.

___ 4. Have you taken thyroid medications most of your life? If yes, score 2 points.

___ 5. Did you lose your periods for more than one to two years when you were younger? If yes, score 2 points.

___ 6. Have you taken medicines such as cortisone (a common type is prednisone) regularly for more than four or five years? If yes, score 2 points.

___ 7. Do you smoke cigarettes? If yes, score 2 points.

___ 8. Are you Caucasian? If yes, score 3 points.

___ 9. Did your mother or father have a heart attack before the age of 60? If yes, score 3 points.

___ 10. Are you diabetic? If yes, score 2 points.

___ 11. Is your cholesterol level above 240? If yes, score 2 points.

___ 12. Do you rarely exercise? If yes, score 2 points.

___ 13. Are you having night sweats where you are drenched and can't sleep? If yes, score 3 points.

___ 14. Do you have incredible out-of-character mood swings? If yes, score 3 points.

___ 15. Do you have vaginal rawness, dryness, and soreness most of the time? If yes, score 3 points.

___ 16. Do you not even consider sexual intercourse because it is so painful? If yes, score 3 points.

___ 17. Have you lost all your sexual interest even though you wish you hadn't? If yes, score 3 points.

___ 18. Did your mother have osteoporosis that either required special treatment or resulted in a bone fracture? If yes, score 3 points.

___ 19. Are you more than 40 years of age? If yes, score 2 points.

___ 20. Have you not had a period for more than 6 months? If yes, score 2 points.

INTERPRETING YOUR SCORE

Tally your score and match it to the category below:

0–15   This score indicates you have a risk of diseases associated with the lack of female sex hormones. Make your physician aware of this before taking estrogen replacement therapy.

16–30   This score implies a greater risk for diseases associated with a lack of the sex hormones. You should seriously consider estrogen replacement therapy.

20 or more   You should consult your doctor and discuss benefits and risks of hormone therapy.

Some of the risks of hormone (estrogen) therapy are increased if you have some of the following:

◆ A precancerous breast condition or immediate family members with breast cancer, colon cancer, ovarian cancer, uterine cancer
◆ Drink more than three or four alcoholic drinks a day
◆ Phlebitis, liver disease, lupus erythematosus, asthma, gall-bladder problems, endometriosis, fibroids, sore and lumpy breasts, migraines, and stroke

Male Sex Factor

Men do not experience the dramatic decline in their sex hormones that women do. Indeed, until twenty years ago the fact that men experience a sex hormone decline was not recognized by the medical (largely male) establishment. Now we know better. While there are no tightly defined age brackets for the beginning of the male hormone decline, as with menopause, andropause is starting to be recognized.

The male sex hormone decline begins in the late teens but does not impact men dramatically until their forties or fifties. While not as severe, sexual hormonal decline varies much more among men than women. It is estimated that about 20 percent of men in their forties are deficient in testosterone.

Testosterone is essential for men to maintain their youthful vigor. Testosterone not only controls the sex drive but maintains muscles, skin elasticity, and strong bones. It promotes a sense of vitality and well-being. Athletes take it illegally to increase strength and endurance.

Interestingly, a testosterone deficiency is *not* strongly associated with impotence, which is also known as erectile dysfunction. About 25 million American men suffer some degree of impotence, but that doesn't necessarily point to a testosterone deficiency. More often impotence is psychogenic (psychological factors) or the result of other non-sex-hormonal factors, including vascular conditions, heart diseases, hypertension, diabetes, insulin resistance, certain medications, surgery, recreational drug use, drug abuse, smoking, alcoholism, and lack of physical conditioning.

One of the differences in the way men and women age is that while women experience a decline in all their sex hormones, estrogen as well as testosterone, men experience only a decline in testosterone. Their estrogen levels do not decline, they increase. In fact, the average fifty-year-old man will have more estrogen than his female counterpart (unless she takes hormonal replacement therapy). Why do men need estrogen? In growing boys it is needed to complete the growth of bones, and in mature men it prevents bone loss. The main source of estrogen in men is from the aromatization of testosterone.

Women need a small supply of testosterone to stimulate their sex drive and keep their bones and muscles firm; men need a small supply of estrogen to keep the brain's neurotransmitter systems, especially the acetylcholine, working properly. Too much estrogen in men—that is, in relation to testosterone—can lead to weak muscles, enlarged breast tissue (gynecomastia), obesity, depressed sexual drive, and rheumatological connective tissue disorders.

Prostate diseases start to manifest as the male hormones decline and estrogens rise with aging, usually from age forty onward. It has been estimated that between 50 to 70 percent of men in Western countries will get some degree of prostate cancer by the age of seventy. It is during this period of an increased *ratio* of estrogen to testosterone that prostate problems begin to multiply. This is counter to the popular notion that it is *only* the male hormones that lead to prostatic hypertrophy and cancer. If this were the case, then young men ages eighteen to twenty, at the peak of testosterone production, would be getting prostate diseases.

When estrogen is given to men in the absence of a male sex hormone, it has a stimulatory effect on the prostate, which in animal studies was *not* cancerous. When given in concert with testosterone, estrogen seems to synergize with the male sex hormone to stimulate prostate growth and cancer. These studies suggest that as estrogen breaks down, it produces 4-hydroxy estradiol and other products that are a source of free radicals in the prostate.

The key to protecting both prostate and breast tissue from abnormal growth—tissues in which estrogens play a role—is diet and certain supplements. The "magic soybean" appears to give protection to both men and women by its estrogen-regulating and -modulating effects. Other nutrients/supplements that may provide protection or "reverse" some of the DNA damage in the prostate include vitamin E, tomatoes (as a rich source of lycopene), selenium, and others. (See chapter 15 for more information on these substances.)

Like estrogen, testosterone is available only with a doctor's prescription. The good news, though, is that where previously it could be administered only through injection and under-the-skin implantation, testosterone is now available in easy-to-use patches, compounded gels and lozenges, and oral tablets. Available in Canada and Europe is an oral form called testosterone undecanoate and a sublingual form called sublingual T cyclodextrin (SLT), which is under study in the United States. These preparations need to be taken two to three times a day.

Testosterone production can be promoted in other ways not involving drugs. It is possible to stimulate testosterone production with weight-resistance exercises that are intense, brief, and do not cause you to become totally exhausted or depleted. Consult Anti-aging Exercises in the appendix for instructions about how to use these safely.

Are you a candidate for testosterone replacement therapy? The following questionnaire will help you to determine whether you have a sex hormone decline that needs to be addressed by you and your physician. Answer each question to the best of your ability. If the answer is no, score 0 points.

MALE SEX FACTOR QUESTIONNAIRE

___ 1. Are your testicles becoming smaller and softer? If yes, score 2 points.

___ 2. Do you drink more than 3 alcoholic beverages nightly? If yes, score 2 points.

___ 3. Have you noticed a decline of sexual interest, fantasies, and ideas even though you would like to have sex? If yes, score 1 point.

___ 4. Do you feel a general decline in your sense of well-being and feel mildly depressed? If yes, score 1 point.

___ 5. Are you more weepy and emotional than ever before? If yes, score 1 point.

___ 6. Is it harder for you to put on muscle despite hard training, a good diet, and a stress-controlled lifestyle when compared to other men about your age and lifestyle? If yes, score 2 points.

___ 7. Have you ever used anabolic steroid hormones? If yes, score 3 points.

___ 8. Have you ever had hepatitis or a bad liver? If yes, score 1 point.

___ 9. Were any of the men in your family ever treated for osteoporosis? If yes, score 3 points.

___ 10. Have you ever been told you have a low sperm count? If yes, score 2 points.

___ 11. Have you ever been or are you now a chronic smoker? If yes, score 2 points.

___ 12. Do you experience a decline of strength or frequency of erections compared to a year ago? If yes, score 1 point.

___ 13. Have you been on thyroid replacement therapy most of your life? If yes, score 2 points.

___ 14. Are you losing pubic or facial hair? If yes, score 3 points.

___ 15. Have you regularly been using a cortisone type of medication (such as prednisone, Kenalog, dexamethasone) for more than 5 years? If yes, score 2 points.

___ 16. Is your memory becoming fuzzy? If yes, score 1 point.

___ 17. Is your belly much wider than your hips, but the rest of your body is not fat? If yes, score 2 points.

___ 18. Are you super-obese all over your body? If yes, score 3 points.

INTERPRETING YOUR SCORE

0–10   You probably don't have a testosterone deficiency.

11–20   You may have a testosterone deficiency. Ask your physician for a hormone evaluation.

21 or more   You have signs that you are experiencing a testosterone deficiency. Discuss hormone evaluation and replacement with your physician.

Caution: Men with any of the following conditions are at higher risk for afflictions associated with testosterone replacement therapy, including prostate tumors, reduced HDL (good) cholesterol, and decreased sperm production:

1. Diabetes
2. Premature heart disease in family members
3. Enlarged or precancerous prostate gland
4. History of breast tissue growth known as gynecomastia
5. Prostate cancer
6. Liver disease
7. Low HDL cholesterol levels
8. A blood disease called polycythemia in which red blood cells increase to dangerously high levels.
9. Obstructive sleep apnea

DHEA: Proceed with Caution

DHEA (dehydroepiandrosterone), a hormone produced by the adrenal gland and available as an over-the-counter supplement, is increasingly being used as a pseudo-sex hormone. *Caveat emptor.* The body uses DHEA to make estrogen and testosterone, and, like testosterone, DHEA could promote libido and muscularity. DHEA could be a way of boosting testosterone and dihydrotestosterone in your sex hormone equation. Long-term human studies have not been done, and the use of mega-doses by the public with no medical supervision is a scary scenario.

The danger of self-prescribing DHEA is that it can be counterproductive. Rather than promoting testosterone levels, with some men DHEA can actually increase the levels of estrogen or increase their testosterone levels beyond a safe level—where it could lead to an increased risk of prostate cancer. Menopausal and premenopausal women who take DHEA risk an increased chance of breast cancer.

If you plan on using DHEA, proceed with caution and follow the first rule when using any antiaging supplement: Start low and go slow.

A better strategy for raising testosterone levels would be to take the new supplements Androstenedione and 4-Androstenediol. See p. 198 for more information.

∾13∾

Your Lifestyle Factor

In chapter 11 we learned how being overweight can dramatically advance the aging clock by increasing the production of free radicals. Indirectly, obesity is also associated with pro-aging, life-threatening conditions, including diabetes, high blood pressure, heart diseases, and even various cancers. How, when, and how much we eat has an enormous impact on our aging process.

Other ways in which we conduct our lives have an equally important impact. The drugs we consume (illicit and by prescription), our mental well-being, where we live, and the types of jobs we have all contribute to the aging process.

Increased free-radical production is associated with factors as diverse as smoking, excessive exposure to sunlight, air pollution, air travel, and prolonged excessive alcohol consumption. All these factors are avoidable. No one compels us to smoke, drink, or get sunburned. While air pollution and exposure to radiation caused by air travel are often beyond our control, choosing where we live and, in most cases, how we work and travel are eminently individual choices, or lifestyle factors.

Let's look at the importance of lifestyle factors in another way. We learned earlier that the two diseases seen frequently in older people are Alzheimer's and Parkinson's. Alzheimer's, which is characterized by a severe depletion of acetylcholine neurons, is the most extreme expression of the Mind Pathway aging track, while Parkinson's, which is characterized by a severe depletion of the dopamine neurons, is the most extreme expression of the Body Pathway track.

Perhaps because they are neurologically based, we tend to think of Parkinson's and Alzheimer's as genetic, or inherited through a mutant gene that our parents passed on to us. In reality, only 10 percent of Alzheimer's cases are diagnosed as purely genetic. As for the other 90 percent, scientists don't have a clue. But they do know certain risks or lifestyle factors increase the likelihood of dementia (the most profound characteristic of Alzheimer's). These factors include alcohol abuse, head trauma (being knocked unconscious), and smoking.

Let's discuss Parkinson's. Dr. Robert Sapolsky, a professor of biological sciences and neuroscience at Stanford University, offers the intriguing theory that the ancient Romans had no Parkinson's disease. His evidence? The Romans were extraordinarily detailed record keepers, and much of the written matter of their daily lives has survived. There are descriptions detailing afflictions associated with the same neurological diseases that are common today, but nothing that resembles the symptoms of Parkinson's, that is, tremors, movement disorder, shuffling, small stepped gait, difficulty in starting and stopping movements, and so forth.

Fast-forward a millennium and a half or so, and we arrive in 1800 when the first medical records were made of the disease we know today as Parkinson's. Guess what else was happening around that time? The beginning of the Industrial Revolution, where for the first time workers were exposed to the dangers of heavy metals—the minerals, not the music! The process of smelting iron, aluminum, and heavy metals (mercury, lead, cadmium, and others) creates chemical compound by-products that generate "oxygen radicals" or free radicals. Could it be, then, that Parkinson's is an invention of our industrialized society, caused by exposure to environmental pollution? As further evidence there are clusters of Parkinson's disease sufferers in areas or occupations involving exposure to these toxic by-products. The answer is that no one knows for sure. Parkinson's is probably a combination of a nonlinear or fuzzy kind of genetic predisposition to the disease *and* the environment, and time.

Lifestyle factors can affect the aging process directly and indirectly. Take the example of alcohol. Long-term alcohol abuse—that is, five or six drinks a day for ten or more years—lops ten years off the average U.S. life span through a combination of increased free radical production as well as the increased likelihood of fatal diseases such as cirrhosis of the liver, heart attack, strokes, and cancers of the stomach and throat. After smoking, alcohol addiction is the leading cause of premature death—those who die before reaching their expected life span. And alcohol abuse is responsible for premature death in the United States on still another level: About half of all automobile accidents, the leading cause of accidental deaths in America, are alcohol related.

Americans' addictions to tobacco and alcohol are particularly pernicious. More subtle are factors such as stress and mental well-being. Several recent studies have confirmed the relationship between major depression and pro-aging physiological changes such as memory loss and high blood pressure, possibly caused by excessive levels of the hormone cortisol. When depression was treated successfully, the patients' physiology returned to normal.

Depression has even been linked to weak bones. It was previously thought that patients suffering from depression were prone to broken bones because they were less alert. This would be an indirect factor between depression and pro-aging. But a research team at the National Institute of Mental Health concluded, after studying a group of depressed patients, that their bones were, in fact, measurably weaker because of an increased secretion of cortisol, the hormone linked to other aspects of advanced aging. These patients had an average age of forty-one, but their degree of bone loss was that of seventy-year-olds.

Everybody knows that stress is bad for you. Actually, a little stress is not only good but absolutely necessary. It is a stress response of the mind working in conjunction with our body that keeps us out of harm's way—keeps us from stepping in front of a speeding car, for example. But a cost is paid by the body for this type of drop-everything reaction. Most of the body's normal homeostatic systems (the daily repair and maintenance routine to keep the body in balance) are shut down temporarily to redirect energy and resources to the stress response. During stress there is no time for energy or fuel storage or tissue repair; your energy vault is quickly emptied and redirected to increasing your heart rate and blood volume and to your muscles. All sorts of other systems go on hiatus, too, including the immune and reproductive, and the digestive tracts. Essentially, all the body's anabolic (antiaging) processes grind to a halt. Finally, the body releases hormonal messengers that heighten your senses—you see, hear, and even smell better.

That's a heavy price to pay, but our ancestors undoubtedly thought it was worth it as they sprinted across the savanna with a lion hot on their heels. Besides, the stress condition was only temporary, no matter which way the chase turned out.

The problem arises with a condition called chronic stress. The body can deal with being in an antianabolic, or catabolic, mode for three minutes or even three hours. Serious damage occurs when the emergency stress response extends from a few months to years. Studies with animals have shown that prolonged exposure to stress can weaken muscle and bone mass, increase the risk of diabetes and hypertension, result in memory loss, and promote reproductive and immune decline. Chronic stress also increases the likelihood that if you suffer a stroke or a seizure, your brain, specifically the hippocampal region that controls memory, learning, and executive functions, can be more severely damaged.

With access to the best medical technology in the world, Americans should have the healthiest lifestyle in the world. But consider these facts:

◆ Fourteen million of us are addicted to alcohol.
◆ We consume 20 percent more fat on average than in 1973, despite tidal waves of warnings over the last twenty-five years about the danger of excessive fat in our diet.
◆ Sales of exercise machines rose to $3 billion in 1996, but only one in ten of us exercise adequately (three times a week for at least twenty minutes).
◆ Depression affects 9 percent of American women.
◆ The number of American men who die of lung cancer (57.1 out of every 100,000) is surpassed in the developed world only by the Netherlands.
◆ The number of emergency room cases for heroin addiction increased 58 percent over the last three years.

Are these random statistics or reflections of a society that is on a pro-aging pathway? Bombarded by a multi-billion-dollar advertising juggernaut that promotes fatty, sugary foods as fun, fast, and healthy, is there any wonder why one-third of Americans are obese? In a society that equates money with success, who has time for relaxation? The choices, however, are *ours*. The commercial white noise of our popular culture might obscure the truth about fast foods, smoking, and alcohol abuse, but—to borrow a slogan from a popular TV show—the truth is out there.

LIFESTYLE FACTOR QUESTIONNAIRE

The following questionnaire is designed to help you determine the impact of your lifestyle choices on your aging process. Answer each question honestly and write in the blank the score that best describes your experience:

    0—Almost never applies to you
    1—Sometimes applies
    2—Usually applies
    3—Almost always applies

___ 1. I feel unhappy and depressed a lot.
___ 2. Financial worries bother me a lot of the time.
___ 3. I smoke cigarettes.
___ 4. I drink more than two alcoholic drinks a day.
___ 5. Controlling my impulses to drink, eat, or gamble is difficult once I get started.
___ 6. I don't care much for social affiliations or friendships.
___ 7. I don't use a seat belt or shoulder harness when driving.
___ 8. When I exercise, I usually go to complete exhaustion.
___ 9. I don't have any interest in sex.
___ 10. My work is unfulfilling, boring, or stressful.
___ 11. I feel I lack control of my life.
___ 12. I don't look forward to the future.
___ 13. I live alone.
___ 14. I don't have a regular routine or schedule.
___ 15. My work usually consumes fifty to sixty hours a week.
___ 16. I use stimulants such as speed and cocaine.
___ 17. I use different types of mind-affecting drugs to get through the day.
___ 18. I use downers, tranquilizers, or sleeping pills.
___ 19. I have abused cocaine in the past.

_____ 20. I have been treated for drug or alcohol abuse in the past.

_____ 21. I eat the brains of animals as part of my diet.

_____ 22. I go out in the sun to get tanned.

_____ 23. I drink or eat a lot of diet foods that contain artificial sweeteners.

_____ 24. I eat snack foods daily (potato chips, corn chips, or other packaged snack foods).

_____ 25. I have a tendency to worry for no reason but can't help it.

_____ 26. I don't handle stress well, and when stressed, I feel a lack of control.

_____ 27. I am in a bad relationship or marriage.

_____ 28. I travel a lot and fly across different time zones six or more times a year.

_____ 29. I live in an area that has around it a high level of pollution, either noise, air, or water.

_____ 30. I don't take vitamins or other health supplements.

_____ 31. I eat two or less fresh fruits or vegetables a day.

_____ 32. I regularly eat (at least three to four times a week) French fries, doughnuts, pastries, or fast foods.

_____ 33. I hardly ever eat fish.

_____ 34. I am often exposed to cleaning solvents, pesticides, or other toxic chemicals.

_____ 35. I have had head trauma with a loss of consciousness for more than one or two minutes.

_____ 36. I take iron supplements or they are part of my multivitamin even though I have not been medically diagnosed as anemic.

_____ 37. My sleep is not deep, and I wake up frequently.

_____ 38. In the morning when I wake up, I generally do not feel rested or refreshed.

_____ 39. I just don't like physical activity.

_____ 40. I sleep less than seven hours a night.

_____ 41. Generally, I don't eat breakfast.

_____ 42. My weight is more than 20 percent over what it should be.

_____ 43. My weight is _less_ than it should be by 10 percent or more.

_____ 44. Laughing is difficult for me to do.

_____ 45. It's difficult for me to be emotional and to express my feelings.

_____ 46. I get upset easily if I have to wait in line for anything.

___ 47. The habits and circumstances of people around me tend to irritate me a lot.

HOW TO INTERPRET YOUR SCORE
Now tally the points and find your score below:

40 or below   Low Aging Track: Not bad! You're adapting well to the choices you've made in life, which by and large are healthy. Pinpoint the areas in your life that need fine-tuning by reviewing the questions. Your Personal Antiaging Regimen will be the foundation for continued good health as you age.

41–80   Medium Aging Track: You're on the right path, but you need help. You're stressed out, but at least you know that and are looking for new ways to cope with it. Some frustration outlets could include deep-sea fishing, singing, dancing, and mind/body exercises.

Chances are you are indulging in at least one of the major preventable causes of advanced aging: smoking, drug abuse (alcohol, tranquilizers, cocaine, and others), and poor eating habits. Follow your Pathway recommendations but at the lower to middle part of the intervention scale regarding supplements and diet. You probably don't require medication but, rather, volitional and cognitive understanding of your behaviors along with diet, supplement, and exercise support. The specifics are determined by your Pathway.

Are you exercising adequately? If necessary, join a gym and begin managing your time so that both exercise and relaxation or meditation are a regular part of weekly activities. Review the questions to determine which areas need greater attention. Follow the prescriptive advice in your Pathway chapter and in the chapters on energy and sex factors.

81 or more   Advanced Aging Track: You've seen the enemy, and the enemy is you. Your lifestyle choices and reaction patterns to circumstances around you are seriously accelerating your aging. Your score indicates that you are unhappy about major aspects of your life (perhaps even depressed) and have a style of not handling stress well, which contributes to aging. You need a method for coping or dealing with your stress more successfully and in a fashion that does not age you. See the sidebar in this chapter on "Six Anti-aging Lifestyle Strategies."

Chances are that you are fueling one or more of the major bad habits that lead to premature aging—smoking, drug abuse (alcohol, tranquilizers, cocaine, and others), and poor eating habits. Look at the prescriptive diets for glucose metabolism abnormalities in chapter 11 for general guidelines to healthy eating. And look at chapter 10 to see if the reason you drink or lose control or can't sleep well and feel anxious may be an abnormally functioning serotonin-melatonin system.

If you suffer from *ahedonia* (inability to feel pleasure) and need stimulants such as cocaine to feel good, maybe your dopamine system needs fine-tuning. Turn to chapter 9 for an evaluation of this system and how to turn it up to give you more zestful and pleasurable feelings in your life.

If you are a constantly restless sleeper, your physiology is experiencing a quiet hell, a continual wear and tear that is grinding down your four main biosystems. See chapter 10 for more information on the dangers and the strategies of dealing with sleeplessness.

It is important that you begin working now toward *homeostasis,* or a balanced lifestyle. Take the Antiaging Cocktail to counteract the increased free radicals you likely are producing because of your lifestyle choices. Follow the prescriptive advice in your Pathway quotient and energy and sex factors.

Six Antiaging Lifestyle Strategies

1. *Avoid exposure to aluminum and other environmental metals and toxins.* While aluminum has been eliminated as a credible theory for the cause of Alzheimer's, the association between Parkinson's and environmental exposure to different metals, fumes, and pesticides is alarming. Parkinson's, as noted earlier, is a condition that is heavily weighted toward being an environmentally related problem as well as part of the degeneration of aging. Any substance or condition that accelerates oxidative stress puts the delicate dopamine-producing neurons at risk.

Aluminum, which is found widely in products ranging from antiperspirants to antacids, is toxic if it leaches into your brain. Aluminum knocks out the brain's antioxidant enzyme defense system.

Normally, a membrane around the brain prevents aluminum and other toxic substances from entering, but with age the membrane begins to deteriorate and get leaky.

To decrease your risk of exposure to aluminum, avoid health and beauty products that contain aluminum, and don't cook with aluminum pots and pans. (Switzerland, France, and Germany are among the nations that ban the sale of aluminum cookware outright.)

More subtle but potentially as dangerous as aluminum is the impact of the various toxins and poisons found in household products, such as bug sprays, paints, solvents, oven cleaners, and other cleansers. What is the cumulative effect of living with these noxious substances under our very noses? There has been no research conducted to answer that question, but why wait to find out? Substitute natural citrus-based cleansers or baking soda for cleaning products made with synthetic chemicals. Dispose of unused paints and solvents safely (in a designated area) immediately after use. Use a fly swatter! Bottom line: You do not want chemicals dangerous to human health living with you.

2. *Eat less animal protein.* Animal meats are pro-aging in the following six ways:

◆ High-protein intake, mainly from animal sources, has been associated with osteoporosis.

◆ Animal protein contains saturated fat that boosts the LDL (bad) cholesterol and total cholesterol levels associated with an increased risk of heart disease and stroke.

◆ The cooking of meat also produces pro-aging substances called heterocyclicamines (HCAs) that stimulate the production of free radicals, which are associated with an increased risk of cancer of the colon, breast, pancreas, and bladder.

◆ Cured meats, such as bacon, salami, bologna, ham, and hot dogs, contain another pro-aging substance, sodium nitrate, which is also associated with an increased risk of cancer.

◆ Finally, unless you've been on another planet for the last two years, you've heard about the dangers of Mad Cow Disease. MCD is actually one of a group of diseases, including Creutzfeldt-Jakob, caused by an extremely infectious virus. Called prions, the virus in humans typically lies dormant in the brain for many years, only to reveal itself suddenly as dementia before killing the victim within a year of its detection. One recent study showed that as many as 10 percent of Alzheimer's patients were actually sufferers of Creutzfeldt-Jakob. There is no cure, and to complicate the problem, standard techniques of eliminating the spread of the virus, such as sterilization and radiation, just don't work on prions.

What does this have to do with eating meat? Prion-based diseases are passed by eating infected meat or meat by-products. There are dozens of documented cases in England and elsewhere of MCD being transmitted by people eating meat—cooked meat—infected with the virus. Therein lies the larger question. Bonemeal, a euphemism for ground-up animal parts, is a meat by-product fed widely to livestock in the United States and Europe—cows, chickens, turkeys, sheep, you name it. Is there a risk of eating meat from livestock fed with bonemeal that might be contaminated with prions? No one knows for sure.

◆ Just about all of our meat and poultry protein sources (chicken, beef, turkey, pork and lamb) are force-fed all kinds of nasty foreign substances such as antibiotics, hormones, bonemeal, pesticide-treated cereals, and who knows what else. These animals live penned-up lives under a great deal of stress. They probably all have very high cortisol levels.

The alternative to eating meat and poultry is to get your required protein from sources such as legumes and grains, or animal protein isolates such as egg albumin protein concentrates, milk-based lactose-free whey protein, or organic milk products. If you must eat meat, follow these strategies:

Avoid organ meats (brains, livers, kidneys, and so forth). Prions mainly live in brain tissue, and toxins congregate in the other organ meats since they act as detoxifiers (liver) and filters (kidneys).

Eat organically grown meats from livestock not fed with bonemeal.

Eat wild game. Wild game is usually low in fat and high in nutrients.

Avoid cured meats.

Eat lean cuts of meat that is low in saturated fats.

Remove excess fat before cooking meat and don't eat poultry skin.
Satisfy your taste for meat but eat smaller portions.
Avoid broiling or grilling meats, which increases pro-aging HCAs.

3. *Deal with chronic stress.* Meditation, yoga, biofeedback, and tai chi
are just a few of the time-proven ways of reducing chronic stress in
your life. There are numerous others. What is most important is to
find releases and outlets that you can do on a regular basis to help
dissipate your frustration, anger, feelings of helplessness, and other
stress-related thoughts and emotions. Seek psychological therapy if
your stress has developed into depression.

4. *Exercise regularly.* Regular and appropriate exercise regimens decrease the likelihood of cardiovascular diseases, obesity, adult-onset
diabetes, weak muscles and bones, stress disorders, anxiety, depression, cerebrovascular diseases associated with hypertension such as
strokes, and many other medical and psychological maladies. It also
stimulates the release of growth hormone, the allover rejuvenating
antiaging hormone.

5. *Make friends and lovers.* Massive amounts of scientific literature
have shown that social isolation is catabolic (pro-aging). Primates,
including the human species, were not designed to be alone. We
live better among others. Isolation induces stress and increases the
risk for virtually every disease. Statistically, married persons live
longer than single people. If you do not have a loved one at the
present time, you should socialize and develop "affiliations" with
friends and relatives. Having trouble finding friends? Then volun-
teer for a needy cause—environmental, social, or otherwise. You
are bound to meet like-minded souls. Last but not least, own a pet.
The therapeutic value of pets in promoting well-being and extending life is well documented. *Even more than exercise*, intimacy and
sexual contact with someone is strongly associated with longevity.

6. *Stimulate your brain.* Here is something to think about: There is a
negative correlation between education and Alzheimer's disease. In
other words, the more educated you are, the less likely you are at
risk for Alzheimer's; in addition, there is a delay in onset and less
severity should it occur. Classic studies with developing animals

have demonstrated that environmental enrichment—lots of stimuli—produces a better brain; the brain develops a thicker cortex
and more complex neurons. But here's the best part: The functioning of the adult human brain can improve at any age when exposed
to an environment rich in cognitive stimulation. That's a fancy way
of saying that reading a book, attending a lecture, or acquiring a
new hobby can keep your mind sharp. The window of opportunity
for brain enrichment is your entire life span.

14

Your Age Factor

"How old are you?" It's a question everyone can answer immediately. I was born in such-and-such a year; therefore, I am this many years old. Whatever number you came up with, though, you are only half right.

In fact, each of us has two ages: our *chronological* age and our *biological* age. Our chronological age is today's date and year minus the year we were born—the number on our driver's license and birth certificate. But this age doesn't truly represent how *old* we are—that is, to what extent our bodies have actually aged. That is what we call our biological age.

What is biological age and why is it important? Biological age is a concept developed by scientists to quantify how an individual compares biologically with the "average" of his chronological age. It's important because, essentially, it's the only measurement that counts. Although we begin our life spans at birth (or conception, some might argue), we age at different rates. When you think about it, chronological age is merely an invention of civilized society. It might be useful in determining inheritance (traditionally, the eldest son in Anglo-Saxon culture is granted his parents' land), but it doesn't guarantee how you look or how you feel just because you attain a certain number.

Yes, there's a correlation between chronological age and biological age, but the difference is so insignificant as to make that number on your driver's license pretty much irrelevant to science. The danger of using chronological age as a true measure of ability first cropped up about forty years ago, with the Federal Aviation Administration. As the first generation of commercial pilots began to enter their senior years, the FAA had to determine at what age a pilot's declining physical acuity jeopardized the safety of his passengers. While recognizing that aging is a debilitating disease, the FAA could not figure out a way to diagnose it. It arbitrarily picked the age of sixty as "too old" for a pilot to fly, thereby losing many perfectly qualified pilots and being stuck with some whose faculties were impaired. The FAA admitted at the time that "the evidence of the aging process is so varied in individuals that it is not possible to determine accurately" a pilot's true ability to fly by his chronological age.

Every individual has a unique biological rate of aging. How many times have you tried to guess people's age, only to be surprised at how much younger (or older) they appeared than their actual chronological age? We live in a culture where no one wants to be described as a fifty-year-old unless it's qualified as "a young fifty." If we think of chronological age as an irreversible condition, then the goal of this antiaging program is to maximize favorably the aging experience through the decrease of biological age and be functionally and biologically younger than our chronological age. The larger the spread between the two, the better (the biological age being the lower number). It is not only how long we live but how *well* we live.

Your biological age is determined by two elements. The first is the genetic hand you were dealt. As in the case of your metabolism, some people have better genes than others and, consequently, age "more gracefully"—that is, slower. The second element is what we do to ourselves by the choices we make in life: where we live, how we work, what we eat, and how much we exercise.

All of us are stuck with our chronological age, although a little white lie can be remarkably rejuvenating! But your biological age can be altered—increased by bad habits and, ideally, decreased with proactive intervention.

There is only one definitive way to determine how effective any antiaging medicine, therapy, or research is. And, unfortunately, that one is nearly impossible to achieve: observing humans over their life span. In the absence of test subjects willing to spend their days as human guinea pigs, growing older under controlled laboratory conditions, scientists have devised a number of "bio-markers" that can measure biological age. Some of these tests are complex, requiring blood work and lab tests. Many, however, can be done at home. And, happily, some of the most precise also are among the easiest to do.

You can determine your own biological age based on a composite score obtained through a series of physiological tests. The following bio-marker tests can be performed by you at home with minimal or no equipment. After taking all the tests, add the "age scores" together and divide by 7 (the number of tests). This average, or Age Factor, is your current biological age.

If you have scored "older" than your chronological age, immediate intervention is obviously called for. Even if you score about the norm, or younger, you can make improvements in your health and fitness. You can decrease your *rate* of aging. Specific antiaging recommendations for each biological age category follow the tests. Plug in the advice that applies to your Age Factor in the next chapter, "Your Personal Antiaging Regimen."

Do these same tests again after three, six, and nine months of following Your Personal Antiaging Regimen. You will be amazed to discover that—biologically, if not chronologically—you can actually grow younger!

TEST #1: VISION

As we age, the lens of the eye becomes progressively less elastic, resulting in a condition called *presbyopia*, better known as farsightedness. We can no longer clearly see objects that are close to us. If you're reading menus at arm's length or have already had to buy reading glasses or bifocals, you have experienced presbyopia firsthand.

To test your near vision bio-marker, you will need a yardstick and a test card. Take a plain white index card and paste a portion of a newspaper article on it. (Don't read the article, we're trying to determine your ability to see, not remember!) Then place the yardstick on a table and kneel down beside it so that one end of the stick rests against your cheekbone, directly beneath your eye. Take the test card and, starting at the far end, slowly move it along the stick toward you. Note the closest distance at which you can read the text on the card (headlines don't count). Note: If you normally wear glasses or contact lenses for *myopia* (nearsightedness, that is) for driving or watching movies, keep them on for the test. Now check your "near vision" ability against the chart below. The result of this test will be combined with the other test results to obtain an average, which will then be used to determine your current biological age.

TEST #2: CONCENTRATION

The association between forgetfulness and old age might sound like a cliché but is simply the result of the loss of our natural supply of a chemical called acetylcholine as we age. Acetylcholine is an important neurotransmitter that carries brain signals. As it decreases, our ability to concentrate decreases correspondingly.

You will need a kitchen timer for this test. The Bourdon-Wiersma test consists of groups of twenty-five small dots. The groups are formed of three, four, or five dots in slightly varying configurations. The goal is to mark through the groups of four dots with horizontal lines and the groups of five dots with vertical lines. Set your timer to four minutes and begin crossing out as many four- and five-dot groups as you can before time is up. Your score is the number of lines you have correctly marked. (Don't count the

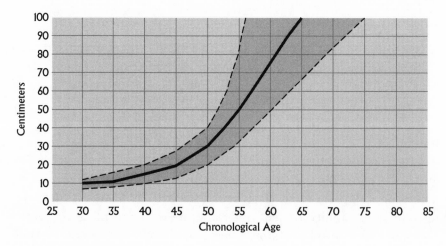

Figure 4—Test #1—"Vision"

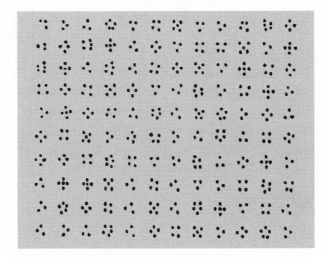

Figure 5—Test #2—"Bourdon-Wiersma Test"

ones you accidentally marked wrong.) Determine your bio-marker by comparing your score to the graph below.

TEST #3: STRENGTH

We grow weaker with age because our muscle tissue deteriorates. Strength is, of course, relative. Fifty-ish Sylvester Stallone can probably out-bench-press barely-thirty actor Johnny Depp. Nevertheless, scientists over the last three decades have determined an

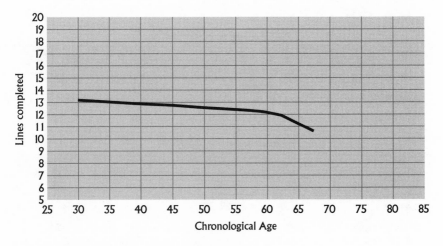

Figure 6—Test #2—"Concentration Score"

average range of how strong men and women are at certain ages. Here's the test: Lean back against a wall with your arms at your sides and a five-pound weight in your dominant hand. (If you don't have a weight, you can use a one-gallon plastic jug filled just over halfway with water.) With your palm facing up and elbow at your side, raise the weight to your shoulder. Perform as many lifts as you can in thirty seconds. Compare the number to the table below. Note: Skip this test if you have any forearm, elbow, upper arm, or shoulder problems; do it later when you are well.

TEST #4: HEART RATE

With age, our hearts become less efficient pumping machines. Cardiac output decreases; hence, heart rate increases to compensate. If you have ever taken an aerobics class, you already know how to measure your own heart rate. The exercise used here is the Two-Step Test. Climb up and down two standard-height steps for four minutes. Try to keep a steady pace. (It's okay to change the lead leg at any time; we're measuring heart rate, not muscle fatigue.) At the end of four minutes, stop and wait fifteen seconds. Now place your index and middle finger on your wrist or at the side of your neck. Count your pulse for one minute. Note your score and compare it to the chart below. Note: Skip this test if you are bothered by knee pain, or do it later when you are well.

	Women (number of repetitions)			
AGE	40–49	50–59	60–69	70–79
Above average	>27	>25	>22	>21
Average	21–27	20–25	19–22	18–21
Below average	<21	<20	<19	<18
	Men (number of repetitions)			
AGE	40–49	50–59	60–69	70–79
Above average	>34	>33	>31	>28
Average	30–34	29–33	26–31	24–28
Below average	<30	<29	<26	<24

Figure 7—Test #3—"Strength"

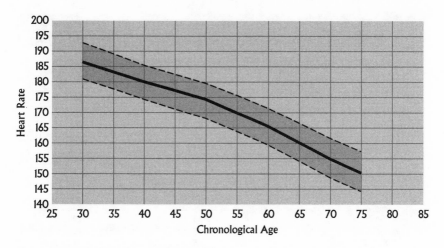

Figure 8—Test #4—"Heart Rate"

TEST #5: REACTION TIME

Reflexes are a classic measure of age. Our reaction time to stimuli increases as we grow older. We become slower at responding to visual and auditory cues. You'll need a yardstick and a partner for this test. As you stand, have your partner hold the yardstick in front of you. Place your thumb and forefinger one inch apart at the twelve-inch mark. Now have your partner release the yardstick unexpectedly. Your goal is to grasp it as quickly as possible. Measure the number of inches the ruler fell. Repeat this test three times with each hand. Add the six scores and divide the total by six. Note your score and compare it to the table below.

TEST #6: SKIN ELASTICITY

What is the largest organ of the human body? The answer is our skin. Physiologically, our skin is just like every other human organ—except that we wear it. It's also the most obvious barometer of the aging process; ask any mirror. While we can't count wrinkles as if they were rings of a tree, we can use skin elasticity as an accurate way of measuring the aging process. Few biological parameters change so dramatically or consistently. Here's the test: Pinch the skin of the top of one of your hands (doesn't matter which) with thumb and forefinger. Hold the skin-fold tight for a slow count of 5. Now, let go, and record how long the skin takes to flatten com-

AGE RIGHT

Reaction time in inches	Men: Body age in years	Women: Body age in years
1.0–1.25	19	19
1.26–1.50	19	19
1.51–1.75	19	19
1.76–2.00	20	19
2.01–2.25	21	19
2.26–2.50	22	19
2.51–2.75	22	20
2.76–3.00	23	21
3.01–3.25	25	23
3.26–3.50	26	24
3.51–3.75	28	25
3.76–4.00	29	26
4.01–4.25	30	27
4.26–4.50	31	27
4.51–4.75	33	29
4.76–5.00	34	30
5.01–5.25	35	31
5.26–5.50	36	32
5.51–5.75	36	32
5.76–6.00	38	32
6.01–6.25	39	33
6.26–6.50	39	33
6.51–6.75	40	33
6.76–7.00	42	34
7.01–7.25	44	36
7.26–7.50	45	37
7.51–7.75	46	38
7.76–8.00	46	38
8.01–8.25	47	39
8.26–8.50	49	40
8.51–8.75	50	41
8.76–9.00	50	41
9.01–9.25	51	42
9.26–9.50	53	43
9.51–9.75	54	44
9.76–10.00	54	45
10.01–10.25	55	46
10.26–10.50	56	46
10.51–10.75	57	47
10.76–11.00	59	48
11.01–11.25	60	49
11.26–11.50	61	50
11.51–11.75	62	52
11.76–12.00	63	53
12.01–12.25	64	54
12.26–12.50	65	55
12.51–12.75	65	56
12.76–13.00	66	58
13.01–13.25	68	60
13.26–13.50	70	61
13.51–13.75	71 or more	63
13.76–14.00		66
14.01–14.25		68
14.26–14.50		71 or more

Figure 9—Test #5—"Reaction Time"

	Time (s) ± S.D.			
Age	Female	(N)	Male	(N)
10–19	0	(4)	0	(3)
20–29	0	(34)	0	(23)
30–39	0.2 ± 0.5	(90)	0.02 ± 0.1	(45)
40–49	1.9 ± 2.4	(43)	1.2 ± 1.0	(19)
50–59	11.8 ± 15.7	(59)	3.9 ± 5.3	(40)
60–69	21.6 ± 23.8	(26)	19.9 ± 20.8	(30)
70+	57.3 ± 31.6	(12)	43.1 ± 28.4	(9)

Figure 10—Test #6—"Skin Elasticity"

pletely. That's the whole test. Now, compare your score with the table above.

TEST #7: STATIC BALANCE

As the brain ages and loses important neurotransmitters, many functions deteriorate. Balance, it has been found, is one of them. This test shows how strong our neurological balancing centers are. Here's how you do it: Stand on your dominant leg, hands on hips, with your eyes closed. Record how long you can hold this position before losing your balance. Repeat the test three times, five minutes apart. Note your best score (the longest time of standing without losing your balance) and compare it with the chart below. Note:

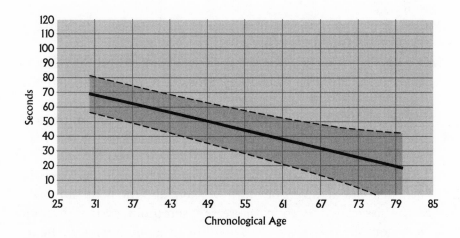

Figure 11—Test #7—"Static Balance"

Do this test next to a wall and in a safe area if you have a balance problem.

INTERPRETING YOUR SCORE

Match your biological Age Quotient to the category below and plug this information into your Personal Antiaging Regimen. This is an overall index or screen of where you are on the aging scale. More sophisticated and specific tests can be done by you and your anti-aging medical specialist.

Age Factor: 35–39

I. OVERVIEW

If your biological Age Factor is one year greater (or less) than your chronological age, then your aging is normal, that is, more or less at the same speed as your peers in the general population. If your Age Factor is more than one year greater—and especially if it is four or more years greater than your chronological age—then early intervention techniques should be applied. Check the section called "Intervention: Advanced Aging" below.

Here are the major changes that occur in this biological age category:

Metabolic: At this age your intestinal assimilation and digestive processes should be operating normally if you have not had any major illness or surgery and have not been using a lot of antibiotics.

Gender: There are no special biological events from age thirty-five to forty that are gender specific.

Neuroendocrine: Your hormonal levels have peaked and have begun their slow decline, including growth hormone, melatonin, DHEA, pregnenolone, and sex hormones. Your neurotransmitter system is also losing steam. On average, the dopamine neurotransmitter cells begin to decrease 13 percent every ten years of life after age thirty-five. For Body Pathway types, the dopamine system may undergo a more profound decline. The acetylcholine neurons begin to weaken, and the behavioral patterns associated with a depressed serotonin system become more entrenched, making them difficult to modify later. The resulting stress produced by a dysfunctional serotonin system produces blood cortisol elevations that slowly munch away at your hippocampal memory and stress system.

Biomechanical: Between the ages of thirty-five and forty your physical capacity remains high, and you should be able to perform exercise and sports activities well, although you are more prone to injury. Muscles and tendons don't have the same blood supply and elasticity as before, but they should not restrict movement. The spine also begins to degenerate. The spinal discs lose their water content and are more easily damaged. Spinal disc herniations and bulges frequently occur.

    The real danger during this age period is what I call "the last chance syndrome." Many of my patients at this stage decide that they must perform a major physical feat at least once in their life, such as a marathon or a triathlon, before they reach the big four-O. Undertrained and with a silently deteriorating biological system in major conflict with their youthful physical self-concept, these weekend jocks experience a multitude of muscle pulls and strains plus microscopic tendon tears, producing tendon inflammation, called tendinitis.

Lifestyle: As we discussed in the last chapter, lifestyle choices can have a dramatic impact on the aging process. In the thirty-five to forty chronological age period for the average person, societal pressures (at least in our society) are brought to bear on solidifying a career, having children, and finding the time to balance family, career, and finances. If one or more of these factors is out of whack, the resulting emotional and psychological stress can accelerate the aging process.

II. INTERVENTION: NORMAL AGING

Diet: Explore switching from an animal-based protein diet to a plant-based diet of protein sources with lots of soy and soy by-products. Soy is packed with rich nutrients, hormone-like regulators, fiber, antioxidants, and many other wonderful anti-aging components, while animal proteins are infused with pro-aging saturated fats. Learn about soy recipes and experiment with tempeh, miso soup, soy veggieburgers, tofu (bean curd), bean sprouts, and soy milk. Learn to cook with soy flour and substitute Nuttlets, a soy cereal, for your regular breakfast cereal. Begin to wean yourself from foods that contain hydrogenated fats, including margarine, fast foods, packaged foods (cookies, crackers), and prepared bakery items (packaged or retail). Read food labels!

Special Advice for Mind Pathway Types: You should add to your regular diet foods that are high in choline and phosphatidylcholine (which is converted in the body to choline). These include soy and nonfat cow's milk, cauliflower, garbanzo beans, split peas, peanuts, an occasional egg yolk, organic lean beef, organic toxin-free liver, bean sprouts, soybeans, and lentils. See chapter 17 for a chart on foods rich in choline and phosphatidylcholine. Animal sources of protein should be naturally grazing and hormone free, from parts of the world that are still ecologically pristine. Wild game and non-farm-raised fish can also be valuable phosphatidylcholine sources.

Exercise: For Mind and Body Pathway types, keep the oxidative loads and stress down by keeping the type, intensity, and duration of aerobic exercise in the easy to moderate range. For Spirit Pathway types, exercise needs to have structure and discipline, and should be done with low intensity, moderate duration, and done frequently for a prolonged period of time. See your Energy Factor score for more details.

Since individuals in this age category begin to experience more injuries from contracted and weakened tissues, it is important to learn some basic sports injury rehabilitation. (See sidebar in this chapter.)

The biomechanical system (bones, joints, muscles) must be maintained in a fluidlike condition to promote antiaging. Creaky, achy joints can be lubricated with a daily stretching program for the major muscle groups of the thigh (quadriceps, hamstrings), buttock (gluteal), calves, neck, and lower back. (See Antiaging Exercises in the appendix.)

Supplements: Begin your antiaging regimen now by taking the Antiaging Cocktail daily and following the advice in your pathway and energy factor regimens.

Lifestyle: The decline of the acetylcholine system begins to accelerate in the thirty-five to forty age category. This is true no matter which pathway profile you belong to. The most immediate result of this decline is a mild memory impairment. To compensate, begin avoiding those lifestyle factors that promote acetylcholine loss and hippocampal brain damage, including stress and certain medicines and drugs.

Here is a checklist of "don'ts"—things to avoid in your life:

1. Smoking: Any amount is pro-aging.
2. Excessive Alcohol Use: If there is any hint of memory impairment, alcohol use has to be stopped immediately. There are better ways of getting the antioxidant effect of red wine, such as from purple or red grapes and grape seed extract. If your memory is intact, more than two glasses of wine or cocktails daily is pro-aging.
3. Anticholinergic Drugs: Avoid these if at all possible, including Transdermscop (a skin patch that prevents nausea and seasickness), the tricyclic types of antidepressants (Elavil, Pamelor, Sinequan, Tofranil), Flexeril (a muscle relaxer), Donnatal, Bentyl, Probanthine (to decrease gut irritation and spasm), and others.
4. SSRI types of drugs: If you have a high Mind Pathway score, avoid taking Prozac, Zoloft, Paxil, Pondomin, Redux, and other SSRIs.
5. Diuretics (water pills).
6. Sleeping/Antianxiety Pills: These include Halcion, Valium, and Valium-based drugs (Ativan, Xanax, Restoril, and Serax).
7. Cortisone-containing Preparations: If you have a high Mind Pathway score, avoid taking prednisone, dexamethasone, Celestone, Kenalog, and others containing cortisone.
8. Aspartame (artificial sweeteners such as Equal and NutraSweet).
9. Exposure to Aluminum and Other Heavy Metals: Don't take supplements with iron. Avoid over-the-counter remedies that contain aluminum, including many (but not all) varieties of toothpaste, antiperspirants, aspirin compounds, and antacids. Avoid cooking with aluminum pots and pans.
10. Chronic Stress.
11. Chronic Allergies: Try to control chronic allergic conditions by identifying the allergy and eliminating the cause rather than constantly treating the symptom.
12. Air and Water Pollution: Drink bottled water. Avoid exercising near exhaust fumes.

13. Excessive Ultraviolet Exposure: A little sun is good. Getting sunburned is always bad (pro-aging).
14. Any Trauma to the Head: Boxing is a current sports trend. Don't do it. "Headers" in soccer also contribute to brain injury. Excessive blows to the head cause brain inflammation and trigger brain cell degeneration, especially affecting the memory system.
15. Indoor Pollutants: Limit your exposure to household and building products containing toxic chemicals. Substitute natural-based products whenever possible.

III. INTERVENTION: ADVANCED AGING

This section is for those whose Age Factor was three or more years greater than their chronological age or whose Mind Pathway or Body Pathway score was greater than 76 points on your combined Mind-Body-Spirit Aging Score (pp. 90–91).

Mind Pathway: If you have a poor Mind Pathway score at this relatively early chronological age, then chances are you will get worse without immediate intervention. Begin by following the regimen of supplements, exercise, and diet outlined in your pathway chapter and in this chapter. If the diet and supplements over a three-month period do not improve your Mind Pathway score, then see a knowledgeable medical consultant about beginning a program with some of the newer brain-activating supplements, including ginkgo biloba, acetyl L-carnitine, and phosphatidylserine, and the drugs recommended in the Mind Pathway regimen.

Body Pathway: If you have a poor Body Pathway score so early in life, then you likely have lifestyle factors that are decreasing your dopamine-producing brain cells. Here is a list of items to avoid:

1. all contact with pesticides, particularly the type used in farming
2. well water in rural farming areas
3. cooking with iron pots, pans, and so forth, unless you have a medically determined iron deficiency; don't use iron supplements unless there is a medical reason to do so

4. speed (amphetamines) and other potent drugs or herbal stimulants (guarana, Ma Huang, kola nut)
5. excessive caffeine. No more than two cups of coffee a day. Di-
lute your coffee to decrease the caffeine exposure. Other
sources of caffeine are the cola drinks, soft drinks, tea (even
green tea), and chocolate
6. exposure to carbon monoxide (such as in parking garages)
7. MPTP (a contaminant found in a designer type of heroin)
8. drugs that block the dopamine receptors, including Stelazine,
Prolixin, Permitil, Trilafon, Haldol, Thorazine, Mellaril, reser-
pine, and Reglan
9. very prolonged, strenuous sports such as marathons
10. trauma to the head, such as that typically encountered in
boxing or soccer

To promote your dopamine level:

1. Perform a daily overall stretching routine, such as yoga-type
stretches.
2. Do light, not exhaustive aerobic exercises.
3. Donate blood if you have a high iron level.
4. Get checked for hypoparathyroidism, a condition that can accelerate dopamine decline.
5. Get a complete blood, urine, and salivary profile for pro-
aging oxidants and for antioxidant capacity.

Age Quotient: 40–49

I. OVERVIEW

If your biological Age Factor is one year greater (or less) than your
chronological age, then you are aging normally, that is, more or less
at the same speed as your peers in the general population. If your
Age Factor is more than one year greater—and especially if it is four
or more years greater than your chronological age—then early intervention techniques should be applied. Check the "Intervention:
Advanced Aging" section above.

The most important events occurring in the forty to forty-nine
age span involves sexuality. Depleting sex hormones result in a lack
of energy, which contributes to a cluster of psychological events
that we know as the dreaded midlife crisis. Women enter peri-
menopause, a premenopausal state exhibiting many of the charac-

teristics of full menopause. Three to six years later menstruation stops, and menopause officially begins. Men get stressed as they see themselves becoming overweight and bald, but they are still filled with sexual fantasies. Sexual frustration can lead to impotence.

Here are the other major changes that occur in this biological age category:

Metabolic: This is the age category in which most people are prone to gain the most weight. An increasingly inefficient glucose metabolism results in wider waistlines and hips. Men develop the apple shape of fat distribution while women develop a pear shape. Your body becomes insulin insensitive as your body fat goes up, which may lead to adult-onset diabetes.

Gender: Your sex hormones have not been in so much turmoil since adolescence. Men are prone to hypogonadism (shrinking testicles), which produce less testosterone and sperm, and prostate enlargement. Women are assaulted by the menopausal symptoms, including hot flashes, headaches, vaginal dryness, weight gain, urinary problems (burning and urgency), and decreased sexual desire.

Neuroendocrine: Along with the sex hormones, all the other key hormones are in decline. As the growth hormone drops, skin begins to sag, muscle mass is harder to maintain, eyesight worsens, hair thins, and vitality diminishes. There is a decreased sense of well-being, and the low-energy syndrome settles in. Key neurotransmitters, notably acetylcholine, dopamine, and norepinephrine, continue their decline, affecting cognitive abilities, memory, initiative, and alertness. You notice that you have less erect posture, decreasing sex and other pleasurable experiences, and diminished ability to stay up and party and be fine the next day. You get hangovers more easily with less alcohol from a decreasing capacity of your liver to detoxify booze and other intoxicants.

Biomechanical: The first effects of osteoporosis and degeneration of your spinal discs may be noticed by a subtle outward curving and stiffness of the mid-upper back with a resulting shrinking in your height. Your hip joints get stiffer. Tendons and muscle tissue become shortened and contracted from less blood and nutrients flowing into and around these structures, leading to injuries. The kneecaps begin to creak, ache, and hurt when going up and down steps, and swell up intermittently from too much walking or squatting, for example, when you garden.

Chronological/Lifestyle Factors: Both sexes have major life event changes: Parents may get old and die, children leave home, career choices are questioned. A loss of youth and a realization of mortality can lead to psychological imbalances and full-blown depression.

II. INTERVENTION

Diet: Both men and women need to increase dietary fiber to control weight and decrease LDL cholesterol and triglyceride levels, which go up at this age. Since weight gain characterizes this age category, your diet needs to be modified to reduce calories and make other changes in the foods you eat. Decrease portions at meals and eat more frequent, smaller-calorie meals to stabilize glucose metabolism. Eat more calcium-rich foods, including low-fat dairy products, broccoli, tofu and other soy products, and the bean family (use Beano or other digestive aids for gas control as you make the transition to eating more fiber and legumes). Substitute vegetable proteins, such as soy, for animal proteins, which create more free radicals and contain lots of fat calories and catabolic (pro-aging) agents.

Soy is especially beneficial for this age category. Soy isoflavones contain natural plant estrogens that can help women control perimenopausal symptoms. Isoflavones also help to avoid osteoporosis by decreasing the elimination of calcium by urination. By decreasing bad cholesterol and increasing good cholesterol, soy reduces the risk of heart attack. Isoflavones are phytoestrogens that help decrease the risk of breast, ovarian, prostate, and other cancers. Finally, soy is a good source of choline, the neurotransmitter that is a key component in the brain's memory system.

Sources of soy products include breakfast cereal, roasted soy butter, soy milk, tofu, tempeh, roasted soy nuts, isoflavone soy protein isolate beverage powders, miso, soybeans freshly boiled in the shell (called *edamame* in Japanese restaurants), frozen soybeans, and soy-based burgers made from Textured Vegetable Protein (TVP). TVP can be rehydrated and used in place of ground meat. For a quick source of protein when you are on the run, try soy protein isolate powder mixed with soy milk or juice. Soybean flour contains no gluten and therefore does not rise, but it can be added to other flours for baking and cooking.

Exercise: Exercise needs to be directed toward losing weight and increasing muscle mass. Optimally, you should exercise at least thirty minutes daily, alternating aerobic (walking, cycling) with a weight-resistance program. But any exercise is better than none, so don't get discouraged if you exercise less! If you scored high in your Energy Factor, then a prolonged (60–90 minutes) low-intensity fat-burning program is needed. As always, consult your physician before embarking on a new exercise regimen.

Supplements: Men should have regular checkups of their prostate. Saw palmetto, stinging nettle, and *Pygeum africanum* are natural herb supplements that can reduce the symptoms of prostate enlargement. These two are often combined to make male prostate formulas. For other nutrients, use the Antiaging Cocktail and your Pathway regimen as starting points, but make sure you take the following minimum daily dosages:

- ◆ calcium, 800 mg
- ◆ magnesium, 500 mg
- ◆ vitamin D_3, 400–800 IU
- ◆ vitamin E, 600 IU

Medications: Are you a candidate for sex hormonal therapy? All women, by virtue of menopause, are. About 25 percent of men age forty to forty-nine could use more testosterone. Refer to chapter 12 for information about the advantages and disadvantages of estrogen and testosterone therapy.

Men in this age group increasingly suffer from erectile dysfunction. When we started writing this book, the best remedy for impotency was a suppository that had to be inserted into the tip of the penis. That all changed with the introduction of Viagra, developed and sold by Pfizer, Inc. The drug was approved March 27, 1998, by the Food and Drug Administration and exploded onto the scene. Prescription sales indicate that more than 3 million men have swallowed the little blue diamond-shaped pill. Sales are expected to reach $1 billion by the end of 1998, making it the most successful prescription drug ever.

Viagra is safe for most men—but not all. As of this writing, at least thirty-nine deaths were verified among men using the pill. That does not mean that Viagra was the cause of death. However, twenty-four of the deaths were heart-related, and men with severe coronary conditions and especially those taking nitrate-based heart medications appear to be especially at risk.

The fact that Viagra is so darn easy to use is what makes it so appealing. Take one pill one hour before sex, add a little erotic stimulation, and at least in 70 percent of all men, an erection is virtually guaranteed. Viagra works by facilitating the blood flow to the penis to make it erect. It does this by blocking an enzyme that, in turn, blocks a chemical that allows blood to flow into the penis. The most common side effects are headaches, facial flushing, and indigestion, and about 3 percent of men experience blurred or blue-tinged vision. However, the major drawback is cost. At $10 a pop, Viagra is among the most expensive of prescription drugs. A number of new male impotency drugs may bring some competitive price relief. Among these is a group of drugs, including PT14, Melanotan-II and Compound II, which work differently from Viagra by stimulating a brain-pathway peptide that is important in the male erection. Thus erection is virtually automatic, requiring no erotic stimulation. Right now, these drugs are only available by injection, but pills are being developed.

Another group of drugs in the pipeline work essentially the same way as Viagra but promise to have fewer side effects. Alas, these drugs, whose active ingredients are phentolamine (Vasomax) and apomorphine, do not appear to be as effective as Viagra in preliminary tests. However, they may still prove useful as adjuncts to Viagra. Finally, a more sophisticated version of Viagra is being tested that, rather than including heart and brain receptors, is more specific to sexual-organ receptors.

What Viagra or any of these other drugs cannot do is improve sex drive. Obtaining an erection allows a man to have sex, but that doesn't necessarily mean he feels like having it. A new generation of supplements enhances testosterone, the hormone primarily responsible for male libido. Among these are androstenedione and 4-androstenediol, natural, direct testosterone precursors that are available over the counter and that have proven to be especially effective with middle-aged men. Androstenedione is found not only in the human body but also in plants such as Scotch pine pollen.

Proper use of these and the five other new T-boosters (testosterone-boosting hormone supplements), which first appeared in 1997, is the subject of an upcoming book that I am writing. Until then, the best advice is to use T-boosters in consultation with your physician and to use them in cycles. If you use a T-booster for too long, your body can adapt and lower its own internal testosterone production. To counteract this effect, take T-boosters for four to six weeks, stop for the equivalent period of time, then resume the cycle, and so on.

Female sexual dysfunction, while less obvious than the male problem, has also grabbed, at last, the attention of researchers and pharmaceutical companies. At least six new drugs aimed at women are being developed to overcome the "big three" sexual problems women face with menopause: lack of interest, inability to achieve orgasm, and lack of pleasure. Pfizer, Inc., the maker of Viagra, and Zonagen, Inc., the maker of Vasomax, are studying the effectiveness of their drugs in enhancing blood flow to the female sexual organs. Two other companies, Solvay USA and TeraTech, Inc., are testing testosterone-based products to treat lack of desire.

Lifestyle: Sunlight is a source of vitamin D_3, but as you get older, your skin becomes increasingly sensitive to ultraviolet rays in sunlight. Your skin also makes less vitamin D as your metabolism slows down. Too much exposure becomes pro-oxidative (pro-aging). Use a sunblocker and sunprotecting clothing and hats whenever exposed to the sun for more than a few minutes. To lower your exposure to pro-aging aluminum, avoid drinking canned beverages. Deal proactively with stress in this turbulent period of your life, using relaxation techniques, that can range from prayer, garden work, petting your cat or dog, "cuddling" with someone, creating peaceful mental images, or using Eastern disciplines such as yoga, meditation, tai chi, and others.

Most important, find something that allows you to discharge emotions and frustrations and that swings you back into balance. Each person can find something special to do that will lead to an outlet for daily frustrations.

Age Quotient: 50–55

I. OVERVIEW

If your biological Age Factor is one year greater (or less) than your chronological age, then you are aging normally, that is, more or less at the same speed as your peers in the general population. If your Age Factor is more than one year greater—and especially if it is four or more years greater than your chronological age, then early intervention techniques should be applied.

You are now well into middle life according to the classic view of aging. The patterns you have set up until now will have a lot to do with how successful you can be in your antiaging program for the next fifty to seventy years. Here are the major changes that occur in this age category.

Metabolic: The stomach produces less acid, making it less efficient in absorbing certain required nutrients. There is an increase of insulin resistance and a greater chance of abnormal glucose metabolism, resulting in increased body fat. This is also bad for the brain because it gets its energy primarily from glucose.

Neuroendocrine: Without antiaging intervention at this stage in life, an abnormal relationship develops between the levels of serotonin and melatonin. Serotonin levels actually stay about the same, but conversion to melatonin decreases and melatonin levels go down. Sleep disturbances occur more frequently. Other neurotransmitter levels in general decrease, causing the physiological changes characterized by the Mind and Body Pathways. And the balance between cortisol to DHEA levels begins to slide in favor of too much cortisol, creating a catabolic (pro-aging) effect.

Biomechanical: Extracellular water goes down, resulting in a decrease of total lean mass. The skin around the neck, upper shoulders, and lower back becomes leathery and contracted. There is a loss of range of motion of the spine. Joint pain and inflammation, osteoarthritis of the spine, degenerative disc disease (back pain), stiffness and hip pain are common.

The Senses: Vision, hearing, taste, and smell diminish as the tissue, nerves, and muscles that comprise the sensory network begin to atrophy. The sense of touch remains largely intact, including the sensation of pain.

Kidneys: The good news is that for the most part the body's digestive and food elimination systems don't deteriorate that significantly with age. A colon of a fifty-five-year-old functions much like a twenty-five-year-old's. The one exception to the rule are the kidneys. At around thirty, they start to shrink and are less efficient filters and pumps. As a result, waste products, medicines, and other substances clear the bloodstream more slowly.

II. INTERVENTION
Diet:

◆ Increase the foods containing B vitamins for nerve function. Eat more dark green leafy vegetables, whole grains, peas, beans, colorful fruits and vegetables, and seafood. To aid food breakdown and absorption, digestive enzymes, such as bromelain and papain, and other digestive enzyme supplement formulas can be added as needed.

◆ Magnesium: This natural element becomes increasingly important as we grow older. It helps to lower blood pressure, block free-radical production, discourage blood clotting, and even maintain strong bones. Nuts and seeds are excellent natural sources of magnesium and fiber, especially pumpkin and sunflower seeds, almonds, filberts, and Brazil nuts.

◆ Omega-3 Oil Foods: To keep aging arteries from inflammation and clogging, increase the omega-3 oils in your diet by eating more fresh deep-ocean fish, mackerel, salmon, tuna, and sardines. Limit herring and anchovies because of their salt content. If you don't like fish, take one teaspoon of fish oil or three to four fish oil capsules (1 gram), 100 to 200 grams of algae-derived DHA, or take 1 or 2 tablespoons of high-lignan, high-quality refrigerated flaxseed oil, daily. Lignin is an excellent source of fiber and phytoestrogens. Or crush flaxseeds in a blender and sprinkle them on your food. Use them right away to prevent rancidity.

◆ Prunes: If you can get over the stigma of eating prunes (is there any food more associated with old folks?), you'll be rewarded with an excellent source of fiber to aid digestion. Prunes are also rich in vitamin B_6, necessary for the immune system, and boron, which helps build strong bones.

◆ Fluids: Increase water intake to one glass every two or three hours. Wean yourself away from coffee, which has a dehydrating effect. Caffeine in coffee also revs up your system too much, depleting the dopamine neurotransmitter system. It also can produce anxiety and make your heart beat irregularly. And too often caffeine is substituted for much needed sleep and rest. Coffee, other than relieving mild depression, does not have much nutritional value. Excessive amounts are pro-aging.

Drink more tea. Green tea has more antioxidants than black tea. I often have my patients mix green tea with a pinch of different black teas for flavor and variety.

◆ Dietary Pain Relievers: Foods and spices, such as fresh pineapple, cayenne pepper, and flaxseeds, crushed into a meal help to decrease pain and inflammation. The spice turmeric has a similar effect and should be used for seasoning. Foods high in color and pigment also help fight swelling and pain.

Exercise: Because the spine and the joints can easily get inflamed at this age, a cross-training program that works a variety of joints and muscles is highly recommended. In cross training, you alternate various kinds of exercises and sports activities to avoid overstressing one group of body parts. A cross-training program might include, for example, alternating golf (which stresses the back, neck, and arms in the same way repeatedly) with swimming, biking, weights, yoga, and Ping-Pong. Hint: Swim with a snorkel and mask, keeping your face down to protect your neck and lower back from over-rotating.

To counteract the natural decline of muscle mass, weight-resistance training should be part of your total program, along with moderate aerobics and prolonged deep stretching. Build lower extremity muscles to prevent loss of balance and injury-producing falls.

Mental Stimulation: Memory and attention span begin to decline. Fortunately, the function and structure of a brain can be improved. The following mental exercises are designed to stimulate cognitive functions and may actually increase the number of brain neurons. If these don't turn you on, there are other time-tested techniques for stimulating the brain: Do crossword puzzles; balance your checkbook without a calculator; take a class that requires you to take notes and tests.

◆ Attention Exercise: Clip a block of seven lines of type (the wider the column, the better) from a magazine. Using an old deck of playing cards, write the numbers one to twenty-six on the face side. Now shuffle the cards, and choose one from the deck. The number selected corresponds to a letter of the alphabet. Now find as many words that begin with that letter from the block of type within three minutes. Repeat the exercise with different randomly selected letters.

◆ Brain Reversing Exercise: Write the alphabet from *a* to *z* using your *nondominant* hand. Once you have that down to fifteen seconds, move on to a series of phrases such as those found in a book of quotations; for example, "The conscience of one is the illiteracy of the revolutionary consciousness."

◆ Playback Exercise: Read out loud into a tape recorder for two to three minutes. Play it back and analyze it for pronunciation, clarity, fluency of speech, and accuracy of what was read. Take a break of five to ten minutes, and then record as best you can everything you recorded. Have someone check your recollection for accuracy.

Supplements:

◆ Digestion: If you have trouble eating a balanced diet that includes the foods recommended above, consider taking digestive enzyme supplements available in health food stores. All these aid in digestion and nutrient assimilation.

◆ Bone Strength: A 3-milligram dose of boron daily is recommended if you are not eating a diet rich in fruits and vegetables (at least two servings of fruit and three of vegetables). Boron is especially beneficial to women who are postmenopausal and may be developing osteoporosis and who don't take estrogen supplements. Boron increases and activates the remaining estrogen. Arthritis sufferers can benefit from boron as well. Also, natural vitamin K_1 (phytonadione), a fat-soluble vitamin, helps to build strong bones by binding calcium.

◆ Natural Painkillers and Anti-inflammatories: White willow bark is a natural form of salicylate (aspirin). Grape seed and grape skin extracts, pine bark, and citrus are flavonoids that have indirect anti-inflammatory pain-relieving effects. Capsaicin from cayenne pepper is found in various balms and helps to relieve joint and muscle pain.

◆ Glucosamine Sulfate: For more advanced joint pain and inflammation, take 500 milligrams of glucosamine sulfate three times a day (or about 10 milligrams per pound of body weight) between meals. If your stomach gets upset, take it with your meals. If your joints feel a little worn, use 250 milligrams of glucosamine twice a day for general support and protection. The preferred form is plain glucosamine sulfate and not NAG (N-acetyl-glucosamine). Shark cartilage and chondroitin sulfate are very large molecules and very hard to absorb. It may be a waste of money to use these and other cartilage preparations.

◆ Vitamin C and Manganese: These nutrients help glucosamine sulfate work better and have their own beneficial effects on joints and many enzyme systems including major antioxidants. Vitamin C has to be taken three to four times a day with food. Take 25 milligrams of manganese twice a day until the inflammation subsides (two to three weeks), then stay on a 25-milligram daily dose. Do not take manganese with antacids; they can interfere with its absorption.

Note: It may take four to six weeks to notice an effect of the above glucosamine sulfate, vitamin C, and manganese regimen.

Medications: Are you a candidate for growth hormone (GH) or testosterone replacement therapy? There are tests that can reveal if your GH and testosterone levels are depleted. Have your doctor specifically check your morning testosterone level for:

1. total *and* free testosterone. A "total testosterone" test alone doesn't always tell. With aging and with certain drugs and medical conditions, the sex-hormone-binding globulin increases and will not release testosterone to your tissues.
2. total estrogens, DHEA, and PSA (prostate test for men).
3. somatomedin C (IGF-1) a measure of growth hormone activity.

Women should have all of the above except for the PSA test. Why are we checking for estrogen levels in men? Because with age and more frequently in fat men their testosterone can convert to estrogen by a process called *aromatization;* they start to adopt feminine features, such as less body hair, more·fat around the thighs, and breasts. Alternately, women can become more masculine looking if they don't replace their estrogens. Their adrenal glands make malelike hormones, and in the absence of the estrogens, women can get more hairy and masculine looking.

Lifestyle: Aim for a stable and happy social life and put emphasis into friendship and companionship building. Men especially have a tendency to focus on professional relationships at the expense of genuine friendships and family.

Age Quotient: 56–65

I. OVERVIEW

After age sixty or so, the gap between biological and chronological age becomes less meaningful. At this stage of your life you need to invest two hours a day in physical training to maintain your vitality. That includes physical exercise, mental stimulation, and stress and dietary management. No excuses.

There is a good chance you will not retire at sixty-five, either, because you don't feel like stopping work or can't afford to. Rather than planning for retirement, redirect your energy to a new lifestyle that encompasses the possibility of living well beyond ninety. Maintaining your health and planning for your financial future will ensure that you take full advantage of the incredible developments in antiaging medicine that will occur in the next twenty years.

Here are the major changes that occur in this age category:

Metabolic: Resting metabolic rate declines. You burn fewer calories while resting. More attention to fluid intake is needed because thirst mechanisms don't work as well. Cancer of the breast, lung, and prostate are common during this age range. The digestive tract and liver have had further insults from medicines, drugs, and time. The pH (a measure of acidity) of the gastric secretions decrease as you make less hydrochloric acid. As the use of aspirin and other anti-inflammatory medications increase, so do ulcers.

Gender: Sexual cancers manifest. Men get prostate cancer and women get breast and ovarian cancer. Some men are already victims of prostate surgery by this age and have to resort to prosthetic mechanical devices for sex. Women get breast implants after mastectomy surgery. By now many women are on some type of estrogen-hormone replacement and are trying to find the right balance of hormones.

Neuroendocrine: Some men are castrated because of prostate cancer and are put on estrogen. Thyroid levels decrease. Growth hormone and testosterone levels continue downhill, as well as melatonin and DHEA.

Biomechanical: Many men have already suffered a heart attack, are on cardiac medications, or have had heart surgery. All of this contributes to decreased function of the heart as a muscle. It contributes to your feeling of tiredness. The joints and spine continue to hurt more and are stiffer. The "frozen shoulder" syndrome starts to occur. A small insult to the shoulder turns into a major loss of function and range of motion.

The Senses: Taste sensation may decrease, especially if you are zinc deficient.

Lifestyle: A good percentage of those aged fifty-six to sixty-five have by now gotten divorced or separated, and may have started new families and even have new youngsters who have twenty- and thirty-year-old brothers and sisters. Loneliness sets in and is felt more acutely if you are single and without children or your children are gone. You might join group after group, desperately looking for that special someone. This can often lead to dating scams and unhealthy codependent relationships.

II. INTERVENTION

Diet: Your diet should be nutrient-dense but calorie-restricted and rich in colorful antioxidant/phytonutrient foods and non-animal meat proteins. Mix vegetable and fish proteins with nonfat dairy proteins; you should no longer be eating a lot of animal meats. Taking off that extra ten to twenty pounds will make you more agile and flexible, and less sluggish.

Exercise: Emphasize lower- and upper-extremity strength, balance, and coordination. Build up the postural muscles of the legs and buttocks and the trunk muscles by doing spine-neutral and abdominal strengthening exercises, such as the Swiss Ball techniques. These exercises involve sitting and balancing on a big round ball called the Swiss Ball. Have a physical therapist teach you how to use one, then buy one and use it at home.

Combine yoga and other stretching regimens with deep-tissue massage and postural-integration therapies to break down the tight and leathery tissues accumulating over the years around the neck and lower back, legs, and shoulders. These therapies, which improve movement patterns and posture, include Rolfing, Neuromuscular Therapy, Feldenkreis, Heller, and the Alexander Techniques.

Supplements: As the body's ability to absorb nutrients decreases with age, it is important to maintain an adequate supply of the antiaging B vitamin group, especially B_{12}. One strategy is to use "coenzymated sublingual" B vitamins that are placed under the tongue rather than swallowed. The vitamins enter the bloodstream directly without first passing through the liver. Other antiaging nutrients sold in sublingual form include melatonin, DHEA, and dimethyl glycine (DMG). Multivitamin buccal (inner cheek) sprays are becoming available as well.

Medications: By now you may be taking some type of prescription medicine on a long-term basis. This drug can modify your antiaging program significantly. Long-term use of many pharmaceuticals are pro-aging. For example, many antiallergy medicines, such as the antihistamines, inhibit the brain's ability to learn new things. Many tranquilizers don't allow the brain to process and gain new knowledge and form new skills. In consultation with your physician, try to change your lifestyle and environment to decrease or stop the use of prescription drugs.

Overuse of medication like ibuprofen, aspirin, Aleve, or antibiotics combined with digestive abnormalities associated with this age group can inhibit the effectiveness of other antiaging medications and supplements. But many antiaging medications can now be taken transdermally via creams, skin patches, or gels, and include estrogens, progesterone, testosterone, Deprenyl, and DHEA.

Also read the "Medications" sections in the previous age categories regarding hormone replacement therapy.

Lifestyle: Balance and moderation should underlie your lifestyle in this age group. Maintain a balance between mental and physical activity of moderate intensity. Control stress associated with work, finances, divorce, relationships, and so forth. Invest in some critical self-analysis to look at potentially harmful daily behavior patterns. Ask yourself, "Why did I do that?" when you overeat or fail to follow your antiaging regimen. Ask "Why am I feeling like this?" when you are depressed or sexually disinterested. Budget time for reflection and introspection. Break old habits if they are bad.

Are you encumbered by the past? Create an environment that is forward thinking by throwing away old things that collect dust and mental cobwebs. Dust can be a good place for mites and other allergens to hang out. Simplify and consolidate to make room for new things. Get rid of clutter. Make your environment at home and at work clean, simple, serene, and happy.

Age Quotient: 65 Plus

I. OVERVIEW

Chronologically, you are at the classic time for retirement, entering what has been nonsensically called the "golden years" but that in reality for most are the "rusty iron years." But these truly can be golden with a practiced antiaging regimen.

Biologically, this is a time of immune senescence (decrease) and cancerphilia (increased incidence of cancer). As your immune system gets weaker, there is less surveillance for abnormal wild cell growth. Simultaneously, a condition called *anergy* can occur in which your body no longer reacts to abnormal substances (such as infectious agents) and cell growth previously recognized as abnormal (such as cancer). Much of your genetic material has undergone oxidative damage and no longer has the capacity to repair.

Other major changes that occur in this age category include:

Neuroendocrine: There is an increased incidence of neurological degenerative diseases, including Parkinson's and Alzheimer's, and of catastrophic neurological events, including strokes, brain bleeds, blood clots, and infarcts. Declining melatonin levels and loss of pituitary gland control over your master regulator, called the hypothalamus, results in many aberrations, such as a shortened and abnormal sleep pattern. This can lead to the major hormones being totally out of sync with the body's and brain's needs. In general, less pleasure is felt physically.

Bodily Functions: Overall, all major bodily functions, including waste elimination processes of the kidney and liver slow down. The nervous system, vision, and the other senses are less sensitive.

Biomechanical: Fractures from weak osteoporotic bones are not unusual, occurring especially in the spine after minor falls. Hip replacement surgery is common. Some may need an artificial knee or other biomechanical body part to replace worn natural parts.

Skin and Hair: There is some thinning of the skin, which results in the skin's bruising very easily. Small cuts heal slowly. Skin cancer is common in both sexes. By now many men are bald.

Lifestyle: The loss of your mate can be devastating. More so for men who don't form social bonds as easily as women. Many men die soon after the death of their spouse or loved one. Some men die because they put their entire selves into their careers, and when they end, so do they. Many of my patients talk about how lonely it is to be old and unwanted. Depression is a major health problem at this age, and abuse of medically prescribed painkillers, tranquilizers, and sleep medications is surprisingly prevalent.

II. INTERVENTION

Diet: Out of habit and convenience, this age group tends to eat the same ten to twelve food choices daily. This increases the chance that vital nutrients will be left out. Experiment with different food types and preparations. Instead of mashed potatoes, try buckwheat noodles or spelt (a grain); soy products instead of animal meat; and mustard greens, daikon radishes, and okra in addition to peas and carrots. Steamed foods, rather than fried, are easier on the declining digestive system. Eat calcium-rich foods and read the section on soy products in the "40–49 Age Factor" section in this chapter.

Exercise: Focus on building lower-extremity strength, coordination, and flexibility, to help prevent falls; see the Antiaging Exercise Program outlined in this chapter. While these exercises can be beneficial for any age group, they are particularly important for this one. The program should be done daily.

Supplements and Medications: Avoid "polypharmacia," or the habitual ingestion of pharmaceutical medications, by exploring with your doctor natural methods of treating your condition. For example, natural supplements such as hops, passion flower, valerian root, chamomile tea, and melatonin can be substituted for prescription drugs needed for sleep and relaxation. To avoid the increased risk at this age of cold, flu, and infections, add to your antiaging regimen garlic cloves or capsules (one to two cloves three times a day or one to two capsules three times a day) or ginger tea, made by thinly slicing ginger, briefly boiling it, and letting it steep in warm water. Throw a dash of cayenne pepper into it for more zest. See chapter 16 for other choices for immune stimulation.

Other over-the-counter supplements to consider adding to your daily antiaging regimen include:

◆ Flavonoids: powerful antioxidants that include red grape skin and grape seed extract, Pycnogenol (maritime pine bark extract), bilberry, green tea, citrus bioflavonoids, quercetin, and others.

◆ Amino Acids: the one known as glutamine can be used to promote GH release and repair the gut and muscles. L-arginine is for dilating blood vessels.

◆ DHEA: increases the sex hormones.

◆ Pregnenolone: provides a material from which five key hormones can be made, and is used to balance the brain.

◆ Phosphatidylserine: activates brain cell membranes to make them more fluid and receptive.

◆ Vitamin E: should be increased to 800–1,000 IU unless prone to bleeding. Use the natural mixed tocopherol type.

◆ Vitamin B Group: the dosage recommended in the Antiaging Cocktail should be increased to two or three times a day. Take B_{12} by injection for low urine or red blood cell levels. Take sublingual coenzymated B vitamins if there are liver or gut absorption problems.

◆ Acetyl L-carnitine: protects the brain in multiple ways. Take 500 milligrams to 1 gram or more if you scored high on the Mind Pathway questionnaire.

These prescription drugs should be taken only in consultation with your doctor:

◆ Growth Hormone family of compounds: an overall rejuvenating hormone. See chapter 5 for more details.

◆ Piracetam: to boost mental alertness; used best intermittently.

◆ Lucidril: protects memory and helps prevent cellular debris from collecting in brain cells.

Thin Skin: The skin, the body's largest organ, is especially prone to damage in this age group. Use a loofah-type skin scrubber daily all over to remove dead and sun-damaged layers. Scrub to the point of mild redness to promote new skin—the same principle as a chemical peel except this is a mechanical process. Retin A and alpha-hyroxy acid peels can be done at home under supervision. Always use a sunblocker when outdoors for more than a few minutes. Ginkgo biloba, a natural herb, is good for the blood vessels of the skin. It regulates them by dilation if constricted and constricts where too dilated. The overall effect is to deliver blood to the areas where most needed. But contrary to some advertising, it does not make varicose veins better. To strengthen and stabilize the collagen of the skin and body, use grape seed extract and hawthornberry extract. The herb Butcher's Broom may help varicose veins.

Lifestyle: Make your living space simple and safe to avoid tripping or falling. Keep relationships going, but don't rely on just one set of friends. Build new friendships. Start new brain-building hobbies: learn the piano, guitar, or drums; play computer games and explore the Internet. Keep the brain juices flowing by learning memory games, crossword puzzles, and balancing your checkbook without a calculator. See Mental Stimulation Exercises on pp. 203–204.

The Biomechanical System

The body's biomechanical system (muscles and bones) is one of the most neglected in antiaging regimens. This is a shame because physical therapy and treatment have immediate effects and can be far less expensive and have far fewer side effects than drugs or surgery.

Why is this system so important? Let's use the analogy of a car. The electrical system (brain and nerves) is in tip-top shape. All the fluids (hormones) are at their proper level, and even the paint job (skin) looks great. But it's not going very far if it has a flat tire and the frame is bent. An antiaging regimen is not complete without the spine properly aligned and the joints moving smoothly.

Problems and Treatments

Stooped Shoulders

◆ *Problem:* Most of my patients fifty-five or older suffer from tightening and contraction of the myofascial layers, or connective tissue, around the lower neck and upper shoulder areas, and the mid and lower back. They can feel pain and stress in this area after a long workday of sitting at their desks. If this area is not treated and stretched, the neck becomes compressed, leading to an advanced aging of the neck and cervical spine—the familiar "stooped shoulders" of the elderly.

◆ *Treatment:* For temporary relief of inflammation and pain of this connective tissue, I recommend a regimen of acupuncture, ibuprofen, and antioxidants. But only until the connective tissue is "unglued" can the underlying bony elements, that is the vertebrae, return to their proper alignment. The most effective treatments are neuromuscular massage techniques, including Rolfing, Heller, and Neuromuscular Therapy; combine with an ongoing stretching program. (See Antiaging Exercises in the appendix.)

Creaky Joints and Poor Mobility

◆ *Problem:* A common complaint with aging patients is that it hurts to move. They often mean their joints are stiff, resulting in a diminished ability to move. Short-term use of anti-inflammatory drugs such as ibuprofen are most effective when combined with biomechanical therapies.

◆ *Treatment:* Mobilize and move the joints through manual types of physical therapies that utilize small, gentle manipulations, not the forceful, potentially harmful manipulations of traditional chiropractic. These therapies are usually named after their founders and include Cyriax, Maitland, and Kaltenbourne. Some of these, such as the Alexander Method and Feldenkreis, include an educational component, combining mental imagery and instructional posture techniques. Patients who have had little result with injections, painkillers, and surgery frequently respond well to these alternative therapies.

Diminished Breathing Capacity

◆ *Problem:* One of the most rapid declines of aging is in our capacity to breathe. A sixty-five-year-old typically has much less capacity to breathe deeply and consequently moves a much smaller volume of oxygen through the lungs than a fifteen-year-old. The decrease in vital capacity and forced expiratory volume is catabolic and accelerates aging in all systems of the body. Part of this decline in breathing is biomechanical: the contraction of tissues around the chest, weak muscles between the ribs, stiffness of the rib cage, tightness of the mid-thoracic spine, and a forward-hunched posture.
◆ *Treatment:* Breathing capacity can improve dramatically with deep-massage therapy to release the tight tissues around the rib cage and free up the tight joints where the ribs and spine join, and deep-breathing exercises.

Tips on Treating a Biomechanical Injury at Home

◆ Use ice for any acute pain or injury. If you have a circulation problem or delicate skin, add more insulation between the skin and ice. Under normal circumstances, twelve to fifteen minutes of icing is sufficient. Use crushed ice in a plastic bag or a commercially available cold pack and mold it around the injured site. If nothing else is available, use a large bag of frozen corn or peas.
◆ If you have sprained a knee, shoulder, elbow, neck, or ankle, wrap the ice around the entire area or joint and gently wrap a compression dressing over the ice. Keep it wrapped for up to twenty minutes, less if you have especially thin skin.

◆ *General rule of thumb:* The larger the area or joint, the longer the ice will take to penetrate.

◆ Repeat the ice application every two to three hours if the injury is bad and has a lot of pain and swelling. Stop icing if you develop prolonged numbness or an abnormal skin reaction.

◆ The third day after an acute trauma, apply heat via a bath or Jacuzzi, or with hot towels. Be careful not to burn yourself.

◆ *General rule of thumb:* Even after the acute injury is over, use ice for any acute or sharp pains that might occur. Ice is a good painkiller, so use it liberally as needed. Use heat for the deep, stiff, and achy kinds of pain.

◆ On the third day after an injury, begin to gently stretch the injured area.

◆ *General rule of thumb:* Stretch to the point where you experience pain. Make a mental note. This is the end range of your stretch. Later when stretching, just go shy of this point of pain. As you heal, you will be able to stretch farther without feeling pain.

◆ The last step of rehabilitation is strengthening. Start gentle resistance exercises, using small weights or isometric contractions such as pushing against your hand or the wall. Again, pain is your guide. A little pain is to be expected, but pain lasting into or occurring the next day means you went too far.

BIOLOGICAL AGE PROGRESS LOG

Use this log to monitor the improvement in your bio-marker test results and to track the progress in your Personal Antiaging Regimen.

RESULTS

TEST	1 MONTH	3 MONTHS	6 MONTHS
1. Vision			
2. Concentration			
3. Strength			
4. Heart Rate			
5. Reaction Time			
6. Skin Elasticity			
7. Static Balance			

~ 15 ~

Your Personal
Antiaging Regimen

Congratulations! You've done your homework, and you're about to reap the rewards. In this chapter you will use the information you have gathered in previous chapters to create your Personal Antiaging Regimen. This will consist of a daily and weekly planner to guide your supplements, diet, exercise, and lifestyle regimen—the regimen needed to promote youthful vigor and vitality, no matter what your current chronological or biological age.

Look at it as an educational tool as well. The world-class athletes that I've worked with did not win gold medals or set records without a plan. Their daily training logs, which look much like this one, include meal plans, supplements, exercise, history, stress levels, injuries, competition deadlines, sleep patterns, treatments, medications, and a record of their effects.

To be successful you don't need to be obsessive with your regimen. You can modify and tailor it to your special needs and time limits. But it is important that you *make an an entry every day* in your planner even if it is a summary of the day in a sketchy fashion. When you put something down on paper, you have demonstrated a commitment to being a true antiaging warrior.

Step 1: Supplements and Medications

You will need a pen and paper to compile a master list of supplements. This list will be used the first time you shop for your recommended supplements.

Begin by referencing the nutrients recommended in the Antiaging Cocktail on page 101. Now modify this list according to the supplements recommended in the chapter about your aging Pathway (either chapter 8 or 9 or 10). As you list the supplements, make a special note of how often the supplements are to be taken (once daily, twice daily), which times of day (morning, midday. before bedtime) and whether they are to be taken with a meal or on an empty stomach.

Continue the list by including the supplements recommended in chapter 11 (Your Energy Factor), chapter 12 (Your Sex Factor), chapter 13 (Your Lifestyle Factor), and chapter 14 (Your Age Factor). Be sure to note when and how much of these additional supplements are to be taken and at what time of day.

With your master list of nutrients and their dosages, it's time now to go shopping, either in person at your local health food store, drugstore, or vitamin store, or as a virtual shopper via catalogs or the Internet. (See the Antiaging Supplement Suppliers in the appendix.)

At first glance this list of supplements might seem overly long, but don't be intimidated. You will find that many of the nutrients are combined in one or two pills. Many antioxidants and multivitamin supplements, for example, contain ten or more active ingredients. Identify the brand names that come closest to your recommended nutrients *and* dosages by checking labels. If you can't find exactly the dosages you need, it's always best to err on the side of being low. And don't be afraid to ask for help from the knowledgeable personnel where you're shopping.

Regarding cost, there are ways you can save money, at least on some of the supplements. For example, plain old-fashioned ascorbic acid, vitamin C—without any bells and whistles—will work as long as you don't have an acid problem. On the other hand, acetyl L-carnitine is fifty cents or more for each 500-milligram supplement, and there is no cheaper alternative. For more money-saving tips on supplements (including cost-saving alternatives and generic substitutes for expensive brand names), see chapter 16.

As a rule, direct mail shopping is cheaper than retail, but you may want to visit a well-stocked health food store first just to see all the available choices. Looking at the dozens of brand names for even a simple supplement like vitamin C, it may seem that you almost need a Ph.D. in biochemistry and herbology just to buy vitamins! But don't panic. Once you have done the initial planning, restocking your private inventory is a breeze.

Insert in the day planner below the names of the multinutrient supplements by brand names or generic brands. Some nutrients may be "stand-alones," marketed in pills without additional nutrients. List these supplements using the name of the nutrient as a reference. If a supplement is recommended for more than once a day, be sure to include each time of day the supplement is to be taken.

If you are taking prescription medications, work with a knowledgeable, interested physician who can help you integrate them with your over-the-counter supplements.

Step 2: Exercise

Following the same procedure as above, begin planning your exercise program by turning first to your Pathway chapter. Modify the program by using the recommendations in chapters 11, 13, and 14. There are a couple of general rules to keep in mind:

If you scored moderate to high on the glucose metabolism questionnaire in chapter 11, your exercise program should include low-intensity, fat-burning exercises conducted for thirty to forty minutes at least every other day.

Remember that the older you get, the more you need (1) stretching exercises to loosen up muscles, tendons, and ligaments that lose water content and tighten with age, (2) weight-resistance training to build muscle mass, which declines with age, and (3) longer warm-up, cool-down, and recovery periods.

If you are just beginning an exercise program, it's a good investment to work with a qualified personal trainer in the beginning. He or she can show you proper techniques to increase the effectiveness of each exercise and reduce the risk of possible injury. Having to report to someone for the first couple of weeks can also get you into the habit of exercising. If after a while a wave of inertia washes away your good intentions, go back to the personal trainer or find an exercise partner who can help motivate you and keep you on schedule.

One last rule: Some exercise is better than none. If you can do only a few minutes of stretching one day because of a hectic schedule, don't sweat it (pardon the pun). The most important objective is to keep the body moving and resist a sedentary lifestyle.

Step 3: Diet

Following the procedure used with supplements and exercise, begin building your antiaging diet by first consulting your Pathway chapter (8 or 9 or 10). Modify the diet plan with recommendations from chapters 11, 13, and 14.

Then use chapter 17 to create a series of weekly meals. Each Pathway has its own section that lists many food choices that are especially beneficial for your aging profile.

Keep in mind two guidelines as you build your weekly diet: your overall daily caloric intake and the ratio of the three main food groups: carbohydrates, proteins, and fats (as established in your Pathway chapter and chapter 11).

Step 4: Lifestyle

If your lifestyle questionnaire in chapter 13 revealed behaviors that are accelerating your aging, make a commitment to change them. Maybe cut down on alcohol consumption, begin a tai chi class, avoid certain pro-aging foods, or even reserve more time for socializing with friends and leisure activity. Use the "Weekly Goals" section at the end of the day planner to chart your progress in meeting your new antiaging goals.

Your Personal Antiaging Day Planner

This is an extremely valuable antiaging tool in the guise of a day planner. Fill in each section as it applies to your aging profile, using the data gathered in the book. Not every section has to be filled in for each day. For example, you may choose to exercise in the morning on Mondays but in the evening on Wednesdays.

Keep this personal antiaging planner with you throughout the day to schedule your regimen of supplements, diet, and exercise. You may want to photocopy the planner before filling it in to allow you the flexibility of changing your weekly regimen when the need arises—on vacation, for example. Periodically update the planner as your biological age improves (see chapter 14).

Monday

Morning

  Supplements

    Before breakfast

    _____   _____

    _____   _____

    _____   _____

    _____   _____

    _____   _____

    With breakfast

    _____   _____

    _____   _____

    _____   _____

    _____   _____

  Exercise/Training (before breakfast)

    Aerobic exercises

    _____

    _____

    _____

    _____

Weight-resistance exercises

_____

_____

_____

_____

Stretching exercises

_____

_____

_____

Breakfast

Carbohydrates

_____

_____

_____

Proteins

_____

_____

_____

Fats

_____

_____

_____

Beverages

_____

_____

Estimated calories:_____

Mid-morning

  Snack

  _____

  Stretching exercises

  _____

Midday

  Supplements

    Before lunch

    _____   _____

    _____   _____

    _____   _____

    _____   _____

    _____   _____

    With lunch

    _____   _____

    _____   _____

    _____   _____

    _____   _____

    _____   _____

  Lunch

    Carbohydrates

    _____

    _____

    _____

    Proteins

    _____

    _____

    _____

Fats

_____

_____

_____

Beverages

_____

_____

Estimated calories:_____

Exercise / Training

Aerobic exercises

_____

_____

_____

_____

Weight-resistance exercises

_____

_____

_____

_____

Stretching exercises

_____

_____

_____

Mid-afternoon

Snack

_____

Stretching exercises

_____

Evening

  Supplements

    Before dinner

_____   _____

_____   _____

_____   _____

_____   _____

_____   _____

    With dinner

_____   _____

_____   _____

_____   _____

_____   _____

_____   _____

  Exercise / Training

    Aerobic exercises

_____

_____

_____

_____

    Weight-resistance exercises

_____

_____

_____

_____

Stretching exercises

_____

_____

_____

Dinner

Carbohydrates

_____

_____

_____

Proteins

_____

_____

_____

Fats

_____

_____

_____

Beverages

_____

_____

Estimated calories:_____

Bedtime

Supplements

_____   _____

_____   _____

_____   _____

Summary

    Diet: Total Daily Calories (for all meals)

        Goal:_____

        Reality Check: _____

    Exercise Training (minutes/hours)

        Goal:_____

        Reality Check: _____

    Supplements: Record comments on how supplements affected your mood, energy level, or any adverse effects:

        Morning:_____

        _____

        _____

        Afternoon:_____

        _____

        _____

        Evening:_____

        _____

        _____

Weekly Goals

Diet

    Foods to Avoid

       ◆

       ◆

       ◆

       ◆

    Foods to Eat More Of

       ◆

       ◆

       ◆

       ◆

Lifestyle Changes

    Things to Avoid

       ◆

       ◆

       ◆

       ◆

    Things to Do More Of

       ◆

       ◆

       ◆

       ◆

Sample Antiaging Day Planner

Monday

Morning

  Supplements

    Before breakfast

    100 mg acetyl L-carnitine _____   _____

    _____   _____

    _____   _____

    _____   _____

    _____   _____

    With breakfast

    Vitamin E _____   1 garlic capsule _____

    CoQ10 _____   first half of mixed bioflavonoid

    Alpha lipoic acid _____   complex _____

    Antiaging Cocktail / Plus half of _____   _____

    recommended calcium dose _____   _____

  Exercise / Training (before breakfast)

    Aerobic exercises

    Antiaging 10 min. stretch _____

    program after shower and _____

    after feeling warmed _____

    _____

    Weight-resistance exercises

    none _____

    _____

_____

_____

Stretching exercises

none_____

_____

_____

Breakfast

Carbohydrates

1 cup natural oatmeal_____

_____

_____

Proteins

1 serving nonfat yogurt_____

_____

_____

Fats

1 tbsp. high-lignan flaxseed oil____

_____

_____

Beverages

1 cup green tea_____

_____

Estimated calories:_____

Mid-morning

Snack
1 handful of roasted soybean and about
$1/4$ handful of sunflower seeds (raw unsalted)

Stretching exercises
    While sitting at my desk, I did low back
    and neck antiaging stretch routine.

Midday

Supplements

Before lunch

none _____   _____

_____   _____

_____   _____

_____   _____

_____   _____

With lunch

none _____   _____

_____   _____

_____   _____

_____   _____

_____   _____

Lunch

Carbohydrates

Italian salad with spinach, endive, _____

tomatoes, onions, broccoli, _____

cauliflower _____

Proteins

Small piece of salmon prepared _____

with garlic and fresh cracked _____

pepper _____

Fats

Olive oil vinegar dressing _____

_____

_____

Beverages

4 oz soy milk _____

_____

Estimated calories:_____

Exercise/ Training

Aerobic exercises

none _____

_____

_____

_____

Weight-resistance exercises

none _____

_____

_____

_____

Stretching exercises

none _____

_____

_____

Mid-afternoon

Snack
Smoothie made from 1 scoop of whey protein,
2 cups soy milk, and some blackberries and blueberries

Stretching exercise

_____

Evening

Supplements

Before dinner

none _____   _____

_____   _____

_____   _____

_____   _____

_____   _____

With dinner

second half of calcium dose _____   _____

second half of mixed bioflavonoid   _____

   complex _____   _____

2 garlic capsules _____   _____

1 capsule ginkgo biloba _____   _____

Exercise / Training

Aerobic exercises

high-speed treadmill walking, _____

20 min. _____

_____

_____

Weight-resistance exercises

weight training, 15 min. _____

_____

_____

_____

Stretching exercises

stretching, 10 min. _____

_____

_____

Dinner

Carbohydrates

a veggieburger patty on _____

whole-grain bread with onions, red bell pepper,

alfalfa sprouts, cracked pepper, mustard, no mayo

Proteins

_____

_____

_____

Fats/calories

1 tbsp. flaxseed oil _____

_____

_____

Beverages/calories

ginger tea with cayenne pepper ___

sprinkled in it _____

Estimated calories:_____

Bedtime

Supplements

none _____   _____

_____   _____

_____   _____

Summary

    Diet: Total Daily Calories (for all meals)

        Goal: 1,800 _____

        Reality Check: 2,200 _____

    Exercise Training (minutes/hours)

        Goal: 75 min. total daily training

        Reality Check: 55 min. (morning: 10 min. stretch; night: 10 min.

        stretch, 20 min. treadmill, 15 min. weights)

    Supplements: Record comments on how supplements affected your mood, energy level, or any adverse effects:

        Morning: sluggish in A.M. _____

        energy went up after _____

        breakfast and supplements _____

        Afternoon: more "peppy" after my

        soy-whey smoothie _____

        _____

        Evening: mid calf pain on right side

        overall relaxed good tired feeling

        ready for a good sound sleep

∾ Part IV ∾

Antiaging
Resources

∾16∾

Antiaging Medicine Chest

Throughout history man has attempted to use potions and elixirs to preserve youth and extend life. The ancient Egyptians were superb chemists in this regard, preserving the "physical" youthfulness of their pharaohs (as mummies) with ingredients and formulas that are still not completely understood. Traditional Asian medicine relies heavily on combinations of herbs and spices developed over centuries for their effects on maintaining health and long life.

Today the health-conscious consumer is flooded with a tidal wave of products promoted as "antiaging," from synthesized hormones to roots and dried leaves. What is the difference between DMAE and DHEA? Vitamins B_6 and B_{12}? Ginger and ginseng? These and other questions are answered in this guide to supplements and other products, some of which have stood the test of time and others that are still being tested.

Antiaging Medicine Chest

Recommended Range:

Do not exceed upper limit of range for total daily intake unless medically indicated.

Definitions:

◆ **Essential Antiaging Item (EAI)** means the item is highly recommended for an antiaging program.

◆ **Conditional Antiaging Item (CAI)** means the item could be useful depending on the medical situation. Consult with a health practitioner.

◆ **Antiaging Cocktail (AC)** means the item should be part of everyone's regimen. See chapter 7.

◆ **Not Recommended (NR)** means the item is promoted as antiaging but has questionable value.

ITEM	DOSAGE	DESCRIPTION
Acetyl L-carnitine (ALC)	100 mg to 2 grams, in the morning.	Related to acetylcholine structurally and mimics its action. Acts as a brain antioxidant, stabilizes neurons, and improves nerve cell energy production. Essential Mind Pathway supplement EAI / AC
Acidophilus and other gut-friendly bacteria	Mix recommended amount into room-temperature water; take between meals. Refrigerated formulations have greater potency than those on the shelf.	Friendly gut bacteria. Part of natural flora; has antifungal activity. Used to prevent and treat yeast infections. Helps to heal intestinal tracts damaged by antibiotics, anti-inflammatory medications, and other foreign substances. A well-working intestinal lining is necessary for proper nutrient production as well as absorption. EAI
Algae	Dosage depends on type used. Take in the morning.	A source of carotenes, vitamins, phytonutrients, minerals, and many other valuable nutrients. Carotenes from the Dunaliella algae and others are well absorbed. Indicated for people who have lost vitality or who don't get enough greens in their diet. CAI

ITEM	DOSAGE	DESCRIPTION
Alpha-hydroxy acids	Over-the-counter products contain anywhere from 2 to 10%, usually in a cream base. Increase applications gradually.	Naturally occurring compounds extracted from foods; rejuvenates the skin by removing dead skin cells so that new skin cells can replace them. Doctors use stronger solutions for facial peels. Have antiaging benefit by potentially removing tiny precancerous growths in the dead cell layers and providing a younger look. CAI
Alpha lipoic acid (lipoic, thiotic acid)	50–600 mg	Important for cell energy production via mitochondria; synergizes with B vitamins in energy production from glucose; has a unique antioxidant effect against both water- and fat-soluble free radicals. Used to treat diabetic nerve damage; reduces glycosylation of proteins; increases insulin sensitivity; reduces blood sugar. EAI/AC
Aspirin	81 mg, available in enteric-coated form for gut-sensitive persons.	Acts as a blood thinner that can prevent coronary artery clots and strokes caused by clots. Some people are allergic to or have ulcer problems from aspirin. If not aspirin sensitive, it is a valuable preventive strategy. CAI
Astragalus	250–500 mg solid powder extract (2:1), 3 times daily.	Well-known, established Chinese herb; immune booster, contraindicated if asthma is present. CAI
Beta-carotene		A pro-vitamin A antioxidant. Avoid synthetic form. Obtain from foods such as green plants, algae, squash, spinach, apricots, green peppers, and carrots. Can also obtain mixed carotenes from superfood concentrated sources like the algaes, chlorella, or plant powder mixes. It is a mistake to take beta-carotene as a single vitamin A precursor and believe that you have taken the carotenes you need. EAI
Black cohosh	250–500 mg of dry powder extract (4:1) or 1 teaspoon fluid extract (1:1) 3 times daily	Used for menstrual cramps and in menopause. Has a phytoestrogenic effect. A German formulation of black cohosh is Remifemin. CAI

ITEM	DOSAGE	DESCRIPTION
Boron	1–6 mg daily; for osteoporosis, osteoarthritis, and arthritis, 3–9 mg daily.	Activates vitamin D, which aids calcium absorption and utilization. Activates and increases estrogen. Need to eat 2 fruits and 3 vegetables per day to get enough. CAI/AC
Bromelain	For digestion 250–500 mg with food; for injuries, take between meals 3 times daily.	Protein-digesting enzyme from the stem of pineapple; digestive aid and has anti-inflammatory effects. CAI
Butcher's Broom (Rucus aculeatus)	16–33 mg., 3 times a day	Contains compounds called ruscogins that strengthen veins and reduce capillary fragility. Can relieve the pain and swelling that occurs with varicose veins and hemorrhoids. CAI
Calcium	Menopausal women, 1.5 grams daily (500 mg 3 times daily); growing children, 1.2 grams; adults, 1.0 gram.	The body's most abundant mineral. The least lead-containing and best absorbed are ionized forms such as citrate, lactate, gluconate, aspartate, and orotate. Calcium carbonate is hard to absorb because stomach acid production goes down with aging; natural forms have potential of containing lead; best to avoid forms such as oyster shell, dolomite, bonemeal, and unrefined calcium carbonate. Sources are cheese (higher than milk), kale, tofu, almonds, dry figs, and sunflower seeds. EAI/AC
Carnitine (L-carnitine)	To enhance physical per-formance use 2 grams 2–3 times daily; for energy metabolism system support, use 2 grams daily.	A vitamin-like substance necessary to move long chain fatty acids into the mitochondria (energy plants) to be burned for energy. Enhances use of fats. For general antiaging purposes use the L-carnitine form. For neurological antiaging add the more expensive acetyl L-carnitine form. L-carnitine is used for abnormal glucose metabolism (see chapter 11) to assist the burning of fats. CAI
Carotene family	5–20 mg natural mixed carotenes.	Natural fat-soluble pigment compounds found in dark leafy vegetables, and yellow and orange fruits and vegetables. More than 600 different carotenoids have been isolated. It's important to use the carotene family as a group. EAI/AC

ITEM	DOSAGE	DESCRIPTION
Cartilage (shark)	No dosage (not recommended).	Has claims for cancer and arthritis treatment. Contains a mixture of sugar-protein molecules, one of which is chondroitin sulfate, a series of glucosamine chains. Glucosamine is the pure building block within the different cartilage forms (shark, mussel, sea vegetable, etc.). Glucosamine sulfate (GS is the easiest to absorb. Shark and other crude forms of GS are not cost-effective antiaging strategies. Avoid the crude forms and use glucosamine instead for treating osteoarthritis. NR
Cayenne pepper (*Capsicum frutescens*)	Use liberally in diet.	Chili peppers (red hot peppers) are used in cooking. Use liberally in the diet for antioxidant and favorable cardiovascular effects. Capsaicin cream rubs help relieve musculoskeletal pain. EAI/AC
Centella Asiatica (Gotu-Kola)		An herb containing triterpines, flavonoids, and other compounds. Does not contain caffeine and is not related to the kola nut. Primary use is for skin and wound healing. Repeated topical use can cause skin irritation and possible carcinogenic effect. Tablets, tinctures, and extracts available. NR
Chaste berry (*Vitex agnus–castus*)	Chaste berry extract (standardized to 0.5% agnuside 175–225 mg daily for a few months.	Regulates hormones. In men, useful for reducing elevated prolactin pituitary hormone levels, which can result in depressed testosterone levels. In women, useful for rebalancing feminine sex hormones associated with perimenopause. CAI
Choline from phosphatidyl-choline		Precursor of synthesized neurotransmitter acetylcholine. With aging we make less acetylcholine, which plays a central role in memory. Phosphatidylcholine is one of the best precursors of choline. A high-choline/phosphatidylcholine diet helps memory by providing choline supplies—if the converting enzyme CAT is working adequately to make acetylcholine (see chapter 8). Best gotten from phosphatidylcholine. New lecithin formulas contain more than 90% PC. For food sources see chapter 17. Mind Pathway supplement. CAI

ITEM	DOSAGE	DESCRIPTION
Chondroitin sulfate	If needed, add 400 mg 3 times daily to the 500 mg dose of glucosamine sulfate	Often combined with glucosamine sulfate in osteoarthritis formulations. Most research favors pure glucosamine sulfate. Very little is absorbed and is not recommended unless you fail glucosamine sulfate therapy. See glucosamine sulfate section. NR
Chromium picolinate and other chelates	200–600 mcg daily.	A trace mineral which helps glucose metabolism by facilitating the action of insulin. Found in mushrooms, brewer's yeast, prunes, nuts, and asparagus. EAI/AC
Citrus fruits	1–2 a day.	Lemons, oranges, grapefruits, limes, tangerines, etc., contain phytonutrient compounds—terpenes, pectin, bioflavonoids, and limonene, which can aid in the prevention of cancer and heart disease. The bioflavonoids are found in the inner white part of the skin. EAI
Coenzyme Q10 (CoQ10)	30–300 mg once daily with food and preferably with vitamin E.	Fat-soluble antioxidant stabilizes the mitochondrial membrane, helps mitochondrial energy production, and has antioxidant properties. EAI/AC
Copper	1–3 mg	Essential trace mineral needed for enzyme functions. Highest concentration is in the brain and liver. Excess copper is pro-aging. Mind and Body Pathway types are not to take copper supplements. EAI/AC
Creatine monohydrate (CM)	For antiaging 500 mg to 2 grams per day on empty stomach before and after exercise as needed to boost energy. Athletes use loading doses of 20–30 grams in divided doses for 5 days, then maintain at 10–20 grams daily for 4 weeks, then stop.	Makes phosphocreatine—backup energy system to ATP (adenosine triphospate) in the mitochondria and is the instant energy for muscle contraction. Athletes use to beat fatigue for short endurance events and rippled-muscle look. Is an additional energy source for antiaging; good for vegetarians. Side effects: diarrhea and increased water retention with large doses. Two pounds of steak, herring, salmon, or tuna contain about 4 grams of creatine. CAI

ITEM	DOSAGE	DESCRIPTION
Cruciferous vegetables (Brassica family)	2 servings daily.	Contain sulforaphane, which helps to convert and eliminate chemicals that could become carcinogens into nontoxic substances, which can then be excreted. Vegetables include brussels sprouts, cabbage, broccoli, and cauliflower. EAI
DHEA (dehydroepian-drosterone)	See appendix 5 for dose schedule. Take in the morning; may have a stimulating effect. For doses larger than 20 mg consult your doctor	Over-the-counter adrenal pro-hormone from which male and female hormones are made. As with any hormone, balance is needed. Your body decides what it will make from it and *not* you; potential harm and good. Can stimulate breast or prostate cancer and lower testosterone levels. Other side effects: acne and increased facial hair growth in women. Used properly in low doses can have wonderful effects as part of a comprehensive hormone-replacement antiaging plan. CAI
Dilantin (Phenyltoin sodium)		An old drug used to treat seizure disorders. The smart drug community found that with small doses a calming, mental-focusing effect could occur. Not widely used. Has low potential as an antiaging drug; serious side effects can occur. Tablets, capsules, and liquid forms are available. NR
DMAE (dimethyl-aminoethanol)	100–1000 mg daily; variable individual response.	A compound naturally found in small amounts in the brain and in sardines and anchovies. Enhances production of acetylcholine. Can have a stimulating effect different from caffeine. Mind Pathway supplement. CAI
Decosahexaenoic acid (DHA), an omega-3 oil	100–300 mg daily; from an algae source or fish oils, take with or after vitamin E.	An omega-3 fatty acid downstream metabolite. Indicated for people who can't make DHA from flaxseed oil; necessary for brain cortex and visual function. DHA is a Mind Pathway smart oil for persons with bad mind scores or who don't get results from flaxseed oil. CAI/AC
Echinacea	Use $^1/_2$–$^3/_4$ teaspoons standardized fresh-pressed *Echinacea purpurea* juice 3 times daily or 300 mg. of solid powder extract, 3 times a day.	An immune stimulant that may be good for those who can't tolerate conventional treatments for certain infections. CAI

ITEM	DOSAGE	DESCRIPTION
Ellagic acid (fruits)		Has antioxidant activity and can help reduce the effects of free radicals. Ellagic fruits are also rich in other antiaging nutrients. Obtained from strawberries, purple or dark red grapes, and cherries. EAI
Fenugreek (*Trigonella foenum graecum*)	To lower blood glucose levels use 15–50 grams of defatted seed powder. Variable individual response.	In herb, powder, and seed form, used to control sugar levels in non-insulin-dependent diabetics. May aid glucose metabolism. CAI
Fiber	20–35 grams daily of mixed fibers (soluble and insoluble) in your diet.	If you are not getting adequate fiber from dietary fruits, vegetables, or nuts containing the soluble type (oat bran, gums in beans, pectins from pears, etc.) and insoluble type (apple skins, broccoli, spinach, cabbage, wheat bran), then between meals take a fiber supplement that has a mix of fiber types. (Do not take simultaneously with other supplements.) EAI
Flax	Best oil form is MAP-extracted high-lignan refrigerated; 1–2 tablespoons daily with food and vitamin E.	Contains more than 25 antiaging compounds. Has the highest omega-3 oil content in nature. Contains fiber, lignan, vitamin E, etc. Crush seeds (use coffee grinder or blender) for a meal that can be sprinkled liberally on cereal, salad, yogurt, etc. Keep refrigerated and use in 1–2 days (keep in an air- and light-free container). Flax oils are PUFAs (polyunsaturated fats). Available as seeds, meal, liquid, and capsules. EAI/AC
Folic acid	400–10,000 mcg daily.	A methyl donor, needed for synthesis of neurotransmitters and cell membranes; works in synergy with vitamin B_6 and B_{12} to reduce homocysteine levels. Found in brewer's yeast, wheat germ, soy, legumes, asparagus, broccoli, lentils, kale, and spinach. EAI/AC
Gamma-linolenic acid (GLA)	Approximate dose 240 mg daily. Contains significant amounts of unfriendly omega-6 linoleic acid.	Essential fatty acid group of the omega-6 unfriendly type. Can increase the unfriendly arachidonic acid. Omega-6 is plentiful in our diet (processed foods, safflower, sunflower, soy, and other oils). An expensive oil. Present in borage, evening primrose, and black currant oils; borage is the cheapest source. Recommended only for specific conditions, such as diabetes or multiple sclerosis. CAI

ITEM	DOSAGE	DESCRIPTION
Garlic and onions (Allium family)	Use garlic and onions liberally in your cooking. 1–2 garlic cloves or capsules 2 to 3 times daily.	Allium vegetables include garlic, onions, chives, and scallions; benefits include protection from cancer, heart disease, and Alzheimer's disease. Onion contains quercetin, which is noted for its anti-inflammatory effects EAI/AC
Genistein and daidzein from soybeans and soy products	Eat soy foods daily.	Isoflavonoid compounds are in many soy products. A regular intake of soy products decreases prostate cancer, heart disease, breast, ovarian, and other cancers. It is not advisable to take them separately because how they work alone outside the whole soybean has not been established. Stay with whole soybeans and soy food products. EAI
Ginger	500 mg to 6 grams with food in dry powder capsules or tea from sliced whole root.	Contains compounds that have antioxidant, anti-inflammatory, antinausea, anticlotting, and other positive antiaging effects. Cook with ginger; dine in Asian restaurants. EAI
Ginkgo biloba	40–80 mg (standard extract of 24% hetero-sides) 3 times daily as a treat-ment dose; preventively, 40–80 mg daily.	Leaf extracts have numerous positive antiaging effects: antioxidant, regulates blood vessel action; dilates and constricts depending on vessel condition and need; anticlotting; increases brain blood flow; improves memory. Needs to be taken consistently for 3 months to notice effects and then continued to maintain the effects. Caution: Consult a medical doctor before using if you have a tendency to bleed easily or have high blood pressure. EAI/AC
Ginseng (Panax ginseng)	Extracts standard-ized for ginseno-side content/ratio or the main root of plants 4–6 years old should be used. Start with low-dose extracts or small amounts of root preparation and work up; cycle ginseng use of 2–3 weeks on followed by 2 weeks off, and repeat as needed.	There are 5 types of ginseng, but Panax ginseng (called Korean/Chinese ginseng) is best known. Comes in 2 forms: white-dried root and red-steamed root. Effects: adaptogenic, antifatigue, antistress, immune stimulant, estrogenic effects; may help menopausal symptoms; regulates blood pressure; positive sexual effects in animal studies, very few human sexual studies; improves brain and muscle energy metabolism. Side effects: breast tenderness. Women with breast cancer issues should avoid ginseng. "Ginseng abuse syndrome": hypertension, nervousness, insomnia, euphoria, diarrhea. Most ginseng products in the U.S.A. have minimal ginseng activity, a waste of money; buy ginseng roots from reputable sources. Cut up and cook in a Crock-Pot in water overnight. Drink water extract and eat the diced root. CAI

ITEM	DOSAGE	DESCRIPTION
Glucosamine sulfate	10 mg daily per pound of body weight; average dose is 500 mg three times daily; take with food if stomach irritation occurs.	Chemically, it is the pure form found in various raw cartilage preparations. Easily absorbed and provides the raw materials to build new articular-joint cartilage. Very useful for the biomechanical dimension of aging. EAI
Grape seed skin extract (red grapes, *Vitus vineferas*)	50–300 mg.	A plant flavonoid, called PCO, that is a strong antioxidant (stronger than vitamins C and E). Decreases capillary fragility; increases cell vitamin C levels. Decreases the destruction of collagen, the most abundant protein in the body; helps stabilize and strengthen cartilage of joints. Decreases inflammatory reactions. Chemically similar to Pycnogenol (pine bark extract); grape seed extract is cheaper. EAI/AC
Green tea (*Camellia sinensis*)	3 cups or 300–400 mg of extract	Comes from the *Camellia sinensis* plant, along with black tea; both contain caffeine. Made by steaming fresh tea leaves (black tea is processed) and has less antioxidant potency. Has cancer-preventive properties. EAI/AC
Hawthorn berries and extracts	Use 3 times daily: fluid extract (1:1), 1–2 ml; berries or dried flowers, 3–5 grams; or standardized flower extract, 100–250 mg.	Contains favorable flavonoid compounds that increase intracellular vitamin C levels and stabilize collagen (strengthens tendons, joint cartilage, etc.). Strengthens heart muscle action; may protect against atherosclerosis and possibly reverse it. Has antihypertensive action. CAI
Horsetail (*Equisetum arvense*)	5–20 mg. Don't exceed 50 mg.	A plant rich in silicon. Few scientific studies on silicon supplementation. One study: 10 ml of colloidal silic acid plus facial applications twice daily showed improved skin, hair, and nails. NR

ITEM	DOSAGE	DESCRIPTION
Hydergine (ergoloid mesylate)	Variable—from 1 mg three times daily to more. Comes in 1 mg tablets, capsules, and liquid. Some patients take 9–12 mg per day; subtle effect type of drug; may take 2–3 weeks to notice effect.	One of the first "smart drugs"; its popularity has faded as newer drugs and supplements have come on the market. Modulates/regulates nerve cell responses. Good safety profile. A nonessential antiaging prescription drug. CAI
L-arginine	2–3 grams before exercise or 2–5 grams 30 minutes before sexual activity (always 2–3 hours away from food).	An amino acid. Large intravenous doses can stimulate growth hormone (GH) release and is a classic test for GH deficiency, "possibly" a large oral dose could release growth hormone. Relaxes blood vessels and may improve erectile function. CAI
Lecithin (phosphatidyl-choline)	For neurological problems, 5–10 grams of 90% PC-lecithin; to lower cholesterol, 500–900 mg.	Old formulations contain 10–20% phosphatidylcholine (PC); new lecithin formulations contain over 90% PC. Pathway persons who need 15–30 grams of PC would need to take over 100 grams of the old lecithin to get an effect and would also have problems with gas and diarrhea. See appendix for foods high in choline and PC. Essential antiaging Mind Pathway supplement. CAI
Legumes (peas and beans)	Eat daily	Excellent sources of protein, fiber, and phytonutrients. Proteins derived mainly from whole plant foods are essential for a successful antiaging program. EAI
Lignan from flaxseeds		Rich source of lignan fiber. Can regulate estrogen effects and increase sex-hormone-binding globulin (SHBG) and eliminate excess estrogen. May protect against breast cancer. Vegetarian women have fewer breast cancers. Lignan-rich flaxseed oil is a good choice for perimenopausal women and women at risk for breast cancer. Can decrease the free testosterone level in both sexes by an increased SHBG. Good for men who are at risk for prostate cancer. The best-quality oils are refrigerated in the store, have expiration dates, and are in light-resistant containers. Look for MAP packing (makes for a cleaner oil product). EAI

ITEM	DOSAGE	DESCRIPTION
L-glutamine	2–5 grams on an empty stomach	Most abundant amino acid in the body. Important for repair of intestinal lining and to build muscle mass. Can be used as fuel for the brain in times of stress. EAI
L-glutathione	Raw fruits and vegetables or 50 mg (reduced form), I–2 daily.	A potent antioxidant. It is hard to increase tissue levels of glutathione by supplementation. A popular supplement in the "reduced" form; seen in most antioxidant formulas. CAI
L-phenylalanine	50–300 mg taken between meals 2–3 times daily. Can cause stimulation.	An essential amino acid, it is the substrate from which dopamine is made. Can improve mental alertness; acts as an antidepressant; helps suppress appetite; increases sexual interest. Can be toxic; don't confuse with pain modifier D/L phenylalanine (see chapter 9). Essential Body Pathway amino acid. CAI
L-tyrosine	50–500 mg as needed 3–4 times a day	An amino acid made from the essential amino acid L-phenylalanine. Required for the synthesis of dopamine. Excess can cause overstimulation. Essential for Body Pathway types. CAI
Lucidril (centrophenoxine or meclofenoxate)	Usual dosage for human clinical trials has been 80 mg per kilogram of weight.	Animal studies have shown removal of lipofuchsin (pigment seen in degenerating nerve and other cells). Stimulates the acetylcholine nerve messengers. A Mind Pathway prescription drug; not available in the U.S.A. CAI
Lutein	I serving of a lutein-rich vegetable daily	Part of the fat-soluble, non-provitamin A carotenoid family. Found in green plants, tomatoes, potatoes, spinach, carrots, fruits, algae. Use whole food sources. EAI
Lycopene	At least 1 reddish-hued fruit or vegetable daily	A potent antioxidant that displays anticancer activity. Found in tomatoes, carrots, green peppers, pink grapefruit, and apricots. Use whole food sources. EAI

ITEM	*DOSAGE*	*DESCRIPTION*
Magnesium	250–800 mg daily.	Essential for 300 enzyme reactions and energy production; 60% is in bone and 25% in muscle. High concentrations in metabolically active organs (brain, heart, liver, kidney). Most magnesium is intracellular. Best test for deficiency is red blood cell magnesium, not serum level; Magnesium deficiency is very common. Best form is chelated, including glycinate, aspartate, or taurinate. Found in wheat bran and germ, almonds, cashews, Brazil nuts, peanuts, walnuts, tofu, soybeans, and brown rice.
EAI/AC Manganese	5–15 mg.	Functions in many enzyme systems for glucose and energy metabolism, thyroid function, etc. Necessary for the production of the antioxidant enzyme SOD. Supplementation can elevate the levels of this most important natural antioxidant. Found in nuts, whole grains, split peas, green leafy vegetables, and dried fruit. EAI/AC
Melatonin	100–500 mcg may be enough for some. See appendix 5 for age-specific dosages. Keep dosage as low as possible.	Natural neurohormone that regulates the body's circadian (day-night, light-dark) hormone rhythms. Measure salivary levels to see what you are making. Recommended if low levels are present and you need sleep cycle regulation. CAI
Milk thistle *(Silybum marianum)*	140 mg 3 times daily (use standardized extracts that do not contain alcohol)	The most potent liver-protecting compound known. Stimulates new liver cell growth and antioxidants; inhibits liver toxins. Therapeutic applications include chemical or alcohol liver damage, and acute and chronic hepatitis. Valuable herb if liver damage is present. For chronic problems 3–12 months of use needed; follow doctor's advice. CAI
Monounsaturated oils (olive oil, canola oil)	1–2 tablespoons of high-quality oil in salad, in food, or in cooking.	Can raise the levels of HDL, "good cholesterol." Unlike polyunsaturated fats (corn, safflower and soy) these are more resistant to oxidation and can be used in cooking. EAI

ITEM	DOSAGE	DESCRIPTION
N-acetyl L-cysteine (NAC)	If healthy, don't exceed 1.2 grams per day.	A precursor to glutathione (to make the important glutathione peroxidase antioxidant). High doses (more than 1.2 grams) in healthy people could act as a pro-oxidant and reduce tissue glutathione levels. Vitamin C may raise glutathione levels with greater cost effectiveness. EAI/AC
Nitrosamine blockers		Nitrosamines are produced in the stomach from the nitrates and nitrites found in cured meats. Can produce stomach cancer. Natural tomato juice, vitamin C, or green tea, when taken with meats containing nitrates and nitrites, blocks their toxicity. Vitamin C substantially inhibits the production of nitrosamines. Green tea does the same. EAI
Nootropil (Piracetam)	400–1,600 mg 3 times daily	Used in Europe for many years, this cerebral cognitive enhancer has a variety of effects: increases metabolism in brain cells, protects against damage due to decreased oxygen levels, aids in transfer of information between the halves of the brain, and enhances memory and learning. Side effects are rare at low doses but include agitation, gastric upset, nausea, and headaches. Useful for Mind and Body Pathway types. A drug not available in the U.S.A. CAI
Oat bran	1 bowl of natural unprocessed oatmeal daily	Contains soluble fibers, and when combined with other fibers in the diet, can lower low-density lipoproteins ("bad" cholesterol), raise high-density lipoproteins ("good" cholesterol), and helps to regulate glucose-insulin metabolism. Found in unrefined oats. EAI, part of antiaging high-fiber program
Octacosanol	Sprinkle food with wheat germ, which contains octacosanol.	A part of wheat germ that also contains vitamin E. AI

ITEM	DOSAGE	DESCRIPTION
Omega-6 fatty acid oil	None.	Essential (body can't make it) polyunsaturated fatty acids: omega-6 (linoleic) and omega-3 (alpha-linolenic). Nonessential: omega-9 (olive and canola oil). The "bad guys" are the omega-6 found in margarine and partially hydrogenated tropical oils. Found in snack foods, pastries, breads and other packaged foods. We have too much omega-6 in our diets. Avoid packaged snack foods, and corn and safflower oils. CAI
Omega-3 fatty acid oil	Take 1–2 table-spoons of high lignan flaxseed oil, fish oils or eat food sources.	Helps to thin the blood and prevent blood clots; anti-inflammatory actions help arthritics and diabetics. The fish oils contain the long-chain omega-3 fatty acids (EPA and docosohexanoic acid) that flax does not. EPA and DHA are a more direct source of the friendly type-3 prostaglandins. Found in dark meat fish: salmon, tuna, mackerel, sardines, and herring. Risk in fish oil is water pollution. Eat cold North Atlantic fish. Dark meat ocean fish are filled with Omega-3 oils. EAI/AC
Pectin		Soluble fiber found in fruits and vegetables. Lowers cholesterol levels. Found in plant cell walls. Skins and rinds of fruit have high concentrations: oranges and apples, and also onions. Unpeeled apples, pears, etc. EAI
Phosphatidylser-ine (PS)	100 mg 3 times daily.	A major fat subtype in the brain that keeps nerve cell membranes intact yet fluid. Nutritional deficiencies in B_{12}, folate, SAM or essential fatty acids (omega-3 and omega-6) or brain insults lead to decreased brain levels of PS, causing low acetylcholine levels, memory problems, and depression. Minimal food sources; small amount in soy lecithin. Effective but expensive supplement. Mind Pathway supplement. CAI

ITEM	DOSAGE	DESCRIPTION
Phytic acid (contains inositol, an unofficial B vitamin)	For Mind and Body Pathway problems, use up to 12 grams daily in divided doses; for abnormal glucose metabolism, 1–2 grams daily.	A fiber component; gut bacteria liberates inositol from the fiber-phytic acid. Inositol is necessary for action on serotonin and acetylcholine and is helpful in diabetic nerve problems. Found in whole grains, legumes, seeds, nuts, and citrus fruits. EAI/AC
Potassium	Take up to 2,000 mg daily.	Essential mineral that assists in muscle contraction and to maintain electrolyte balance in body fluids. Increase if there is more loss due to sweating or diarrhea. Essential for life. EAI/AC
Pregnenolone	See appendix 5 for doses. Take in the morning. May have a stimulating effect.	A hormone made in the brain and adrenal gland; declines with aging. From pregnenolone you can make DHEA, cortisol, aldosterone, and progesterone. It is called a neurohormone because of its abundance in the brain and its neurologic effects. CAI
Psyllium seed	1 teaspoon or tablespoon mixed with juice or water, or eat crushed seeds	Husks assist in bowel movements, are water soluble, and may help to lower cholesterol. See Fiber regarding need for a proper mixed balance of soluble and insoluble fiber types that are essential anti-aging items. Psyllium alone does not do the job. EAI
Quercetin	200–500 mg 3 times daily, 30 minutes before meals	A bioflavonoid that has significant anti-inflammatory action (inhibits histamine release). Good for persons with allergies. May inhibit the development of diabetic complications. Antiviral and antitumor activity. A chronic low dose use may help decrease the inflammatory processes of aging. Found in red or yellow onions, shallots, and broccoli. EAI/AC
Riboflavin (vitamin B$_2$)	10–40 mg.	Gives urine the familiar yellow color. Needed to regenerate the important natural antioxidant glutathione and necessary for energy production. Nontoxic vitamin. Found in brewer's yeast, almonds, organ meats, wheat germ, mushrooms, whole grains, and soy beans. EAI/AC

ITEM	DOSAGE	DESCRIPTION
S-adenosylme-thionine (SAM)	Osteoarthritis dose: increase gradually from a divided total dosage of 400 mg per day up to 1,200 mg. Stay there for 3 weeks, then decrease slowly to 200 mg twice daily for maintenance.	A naturally occurring agent involved in many reactions related to folic acid and B₁₂. In depressed patients it increases dopamine, serotonin, and phosphatidylserine. Is a cleaner and better antidepressant than the Elavil-type drugs. Helps make cartilage with impressive effects in osteo-arthritis patients; improves mood and decreases pain in fibromyalgia. Not available in the U.S.A. Side effect: gastrointestinal. Avoid in manic-depressives. Impressive potential as an antiaging supplement. CAI
Saw palmetto (Serenoa repens)	160 mg twice daily (standardized fat-soluble extracts of 85–95% fatty acids and sterols).	Widely used for benign prostatic enlargement. Compares favorably with pharmaceutical therapies; added advantage is that it blocks estrogen and decreases negative actions of estrogen and dihydrotestosterone in the prostate. CAI
Seaweed, algae, sea vegetable	Eat a little seaweed and the green superfoods daily.	Living organisms that contain an incredibly dense variety of nutrients. The super grasses—barley, wheat, and alfalfa—are also nutrient dense. The super greens are algae and grasses. EAI
Selegiline (Deprenyl, Eldepryl)	Dosage is age dependent, from 1 to 5 mg in the morning. 1 mg at age 40; 5 mg at age 60 or more as needed—can be stimulating	Used to treat Parkinson's disease since '60s. Popular with "smart druggies" and sex-stimulant seekers for past 10 years. Widely used with good, safe profile in the 5 mg and under doses. A Body Pathway medication since it blocks the demise of dopamine; useful if supplement therapy fails and/or as an adjunct. Don't use with the SSRI antidepressants and Demerol. Watch blood pressure; don't use if caffeine or stimulant sensitive. CAI
Selenium	100–400 mcg (selenomethio-nine) or from selenium-rich yeast.	An essential antiaging trace mineral. Is part of the important internal natural water-soluble antioxidant enzyme system called glutathione peroxidase, which with vitamin E prevents free radical damage of cell membranes. The role of selenium is becoming firm: it prevents accelerated aging. EAI/AC

ITEM	DOSAGE	DESCRIPTION
Saint-John's-wort *(Hypericum perforatum)*	For non-major depression: 300 mg (0.3% extract) 3 times daily with food.	Inhibits the breakdown of the major neurotransmitters and acts as an antidepressant by elevating brain levels. Do not mix with Deprenyl, l-tryptophan, 5-hydroxytryptophan, or L-dopa. *RULE: don't use other psychoactive substances while on it.* Avoid ultraviolet light. Special herb for persons not responding to the regimens in chapters 8, 9, and 10. CAI
Soybeans	Use soy products daily.	My number one choice of an antiaging food. Soy beans and their products (tofu, soy milk, burgers, textured vegetable protein, etc.) are indispensable as part of an antiaging regimen. Some of soy's actions: antioxidant, hormone regulation, lowers cholesterol, decreases bone loss, decreases cancers. Lactose free, they contain calcium. EAI
Tretinoin (Retin-A products)	Apply as medically directed.	Prescription products that remove old skin and small, potentially precancerous growths and promote new skin growth with less wrinkles. Consult a physician. CAI
Turmeric *(Curcuma longa)*	400–800 mg 3 times daily between meals; take with brome-lain in equal amounts to enhance absorption; liberally eat foods with curry powder and mustard for turmeric effect.	Herbal ingredient in curry powder and mustard. The volatile orange-yellow oil in turmeric is called curcumin. Has antioxidant, anticancer, anti-inflammatory effects. Positive effect on the cardiovascular system, liver, and intestinal tract. Don't use if you have obstruction of bile flow. EAI
Umbelliferous vegetables		Carrots, celery, and parsnips contain fiber, carotenoids, flavonoids, coumarins, phenolic acids. Have anticancer and antioxidant phytonutrients. EAI
Vasopressin (antidiuretic hormone)	Dosage and use varies with each product.	Hormone made by the pituitary gland to regulate urine volume. Smart drug people started to use this prescription drug in the '80s and noted some cognitive enhancement. Not recommended for an antiaging program. Too many potential serious side effects. NR

ITEM	DOSAGE	DESCRIPTION
Vinpocetine	5 to 10 mg a day. Takes 1 full year to reach maximum potential.	Periwinkle plant extract. Increases blood flow and the brain production of ATP. Accelerates the consumption of glucose and oxygen in the brain. May help the brain to store more information. NR
Vitamin B₁ (thiamine)	50–100 mg.	Mimics acetylcholine, needed for brain energy production. Needs magnesium for activation. Alcohol, coffee, black tea tannins, and sulfites destroy thiamine. High doses (3–8 grams) daily improves Mind Pathway conditions such as age-associated memory impairment, Alzheimer's, etc. No toxicity. Found in brewer's yeast, wheat germ, sunflower seeds, pine nuts, peanuts with skins, dry soybeans, Brazil nuts, pecans, pinto beans, and split peas. EAI/AC
Vitamin B₃ nicotinic acid, NADH, Niacinamide	20–1,200 mg.	Involved in over 50 reactions in the body: energy production, carbohydrate-glucose metabolism, fat metabolism, cholesterol; production of sex and adrenal hormones. Different forms have different functions. Nicotinic acid, the flush type of niacin, is used to lower cholesterol; niacinamide for arthritis and diabetes. And NADH, which can have positive effects for Body Pathway conditions. EAI/AC
Vitamin B₅ (pantothenic acid)	250 mg–2 grams.	Needed to make two vital compounds to utilize fats and glucose for energy production. Necessary to make red cells and adrenal hormone. Synergizes with CoQ10, and L-carnitine to transport fat into mitochondria to be burned as fuel. Found in brewer's yeast, calf liver, peanuts, mushrooms, soybeans, split peas, pecans, oatmeal, sunflower seeds, lentils, oranges, and strawberries. EAI/AC
Vitamin B₆ (pyridoxine)	25–100 mg.	Very important for synthesis of neurotransmitters and as part of therapy for elevated homocysteine levels. Makes new proteins (synergizes the anabolic pathway), red cells, hormones, and aids immune function. If taken in doses larger than 50 mg at once, the liver may get overloaded and there may be no rise in blood levels. Found in sunflower seeds, wheat germ, soybeans, walnuts, lentils, beans, whole grains, bananas, spinach, potatoes, and cauliflower. EAI/AC

ITEM	DOSAGE	DESCRIPTION
Vitamin B_{12} (cobalamin)	500–2000 mcg daily; best forms are sublingual methyl cobalamin.	A methyl donor needed for cell membranes and neurotransmitter synthesis; is necessary to prevent elevated homocysteine levels. Vitamins B_{12}, B_6, and folic acid work synergistically. Best to supplement together. Alzheimer's patients often have low B_{12} levels. Mainly found in animal foods: liver, lamb, clam, oysters, sardines, trout, salmon, eggs, and cheese. EAI/AC
Vitamin C (ascorbic acid)	500 mg to 6 grams daily.	Water-soluble antioxidant; first line of antioxidant defense system. Other major function is to make collagen, the body's most abundant protein that holds our bodies together (connective tissue). Also part of immune function and needed to make neurotransmitters, carnitine, hormones, and the utilization of nutrients. Found in acerola, red chili peppers, guavas, red and green peppers, kale, strawberries, papaya, spinach, and oranges. The carotenes enhance vitamin C action in the body. EAI/AC
Vitamin E family	400–1,000 IU.	Fat-soluble antioxidants. Many forms available; natural form is advised. Avoid synthetic forms that have "dl" in front of tocopherol. Highest activity is in d-alpha tocopherol succinate and acetate. For antiaging use mixed natural forms containing alpha, beta, delta, and gamma tocopherols. Gamma tocopherol is an important antioxidant trapper of air pollutants (peroxynitrite) and should be in your vitamin E formula. Recent studies show that 1,000 IU may slow progression of Alzheimer's dementia. Found in oils, seeds, nuts, whole grains, soybeans. EAI/AC
Vitamin K_1 (phytonadione or phylloquinone)	60–300 mcg.	Vitamin K_1, $_2$, and $_3$ all aid in the production of clotting factors. K_1 has special antiaging effects: helps to hold calcium in place within bones. Found in green leafy vegetables and fat-soluble chlorophyll supplements. Fat-soluble chlorophyll is the best source. The natural vitamin and fat-soluble chlorophyll are useful in prevention and treatment of osteoporosis. EAI/AC

ITEM	DOSAGE	DESCRIPTION
Wheat bran (fiber)	2 servings of wheat bran–rich foods and cereals. Total daily fiber required for antiaging is 20–35 grams from soluble and insoluble types.	An insoluble fiber. The soluble ones include oat and rice bran, guar gum in beans, etc. Wheat bran helps bowel movements (increases size and weight); is partially digested to short-chain fatty acids, which nourish the intestines. Increase fiber slowly to keep gas production down. EAI
White willow bark (Salix alba)	1–2 capsules as needed every 4 to 6 hours.	A natural source of an aspirin-like compound, salicin. Used like aspirin for pain, fever, and inflammation. Also contains tannins, flavonoids, and glycosides that could have added possible positive effects; effects are less immediate than aspirin. Don't use if allergic or aspirin sensitive. CAI
Yohimbe tree bark (Pausinystalia) or Yocon		Yocon, 5.4 mg tablets (yohimbine hydrochloride), is an FDA-approved drug for impotence. Success rate about 30–40% for erectile dysfunction. Side effects: anxiety, dizziness, increased blood pressure. There is no control over the level of yohimbine in bark extracts. Yocon used under medical supervision may help some men. Yohimbine bark extracts are not recommended. Its place in treating erectile dysfunction is questionable, since Viagra. NR
Zinc	15–35 mg. Found in oysters, shellfish, fish, red meats. Zinc in plants is hard to absorb. Toxicity with chronic use of more than 75–100 mg per day. Don't take with high-fiber foods.	Is in every cell and involved in over 200 enzyme systems. Necessary for function of hormones: insulin, sex hormones, thymic, and growth hormone. Essential for vision, taste, and smell; important for prostate function and male fertility; aids protein synthesis and cell growth after surgery, wounds, etc. Good zinc forms are picolinate, citrate, glycerate, monomethionine, and other chelates. With aging, zinc needs go up. EAI/AC

~17~

Food Choices

Food is a major player in the aging process. In chapter 7 we learned how eating "smart" can decrease the body's catabolic (pro-aging) process by supplying nutrients that can restore the harmony of the hormone levels that has been lost with age.

Chapter 11 discussed how our glucose metabolism system—the way the body turns food into energy—declines with aging but can be exacerbated by a combination of poor diet and sedentary lifestyle. Left untreated, abnormal glucose metabolism (AGM) can lead to an increased risk of heart attack, diabetes, and other debilitating health problems. And chapters 13 and 14 outlined how some modifications in eating habits can improve the quality of life at any age.

A successful antiaging program must start with a review of diet. What you're eating can actually accelerate your aging. Take a moment now to review your Pathway chapter (8, 9, or 10) to refresh the dietary recommendations suggested for your aging track. Now turn to the appropriate section in this chapter to build a diet containing pro-Pathway foods. Use the calorie column to create a daily menu or meals that do not exceed your individual caloric intake. And use the carbohydrate-fat-protein columns to create meals that have balanced primary food groups.

The last section of this chapter is devoted to high- and low-glycemic foods. If you scored high on the Energy Metabolism questionnaire in chapter 11, this section is particularly important. Wean yourself away from refined and processed high-glycemic foods that exhaust your metabolism with rapid surges of quickly digested starches. A low-glycemic diet rich in natural fiber and color (from red-yellow-orange and dark green fruits and vegetables), which promote a slow insulin response, is the foundation for an effective antiaging regimen.

Mind Pathway Foods Rich in Choline and Phosphatidylcholine

Choline is the major building block for the neurotransmitter acetylcholine. You can find choline and its precursor phosphatidylcholine in many foods, including those listed below (from high to low in content).

Selected Foods	Calories	Choline (µmol/kg)	Phosphatidylcholine (µmol/kg)	Fat (grams)	Carbohydrate (grams)	Protein (grams)
Eggs (Ig), hard/soft boiled	77	42	52,000	5.3	0.6	6.3
Eggs (Ig), scrambled	101	42	52,000	7.5	1.3	6.8
Beef liver, 3.5 oz	161	5831	43,500	4.9	3.4	24.4
Beef steak, top sirloin, 3.5 oz	229	75	6030	11.6	0.0	29.2
Peanuts, dry-roasted, 1 oz	164	4546	4960	13.9	6.0	6.6
Peanut butter, creamy, 2T	188	3895	3937	16.0	6.6	7.9
Peanut butter, chunky, 2T	188	3895	3947	16.0	6.9	7.7
Iceberg lettuce, 1 leaf	3	2930	132	0.0	0.4	0.2
Butter, 1 T	36	42	1760	4.1	0.0	0.0
Cauliflower, boiled, $^1/_2$ cup	15	1306	2770	0.1	2.5	1.2
Whole wheat bread, 1 slice	70	968	340	1.0	11.4	3.0
Milk, 3.3% fat, 8 fl oz	150	150	148	8.2	11.4	8.0
Tomato, 1 red raw	26	430	52	0.4	5.7	1.0

Body Pathway Foods Rich in Tyrosine and Phenylalanine

Tyrosine (TYR) and phenylalanine (PHE) are amino acids that can be found in foods. Both are necessary for the production of the neurotransmitter system involving dopamine. Always use foods first to try to remedy your Body Pathway problem and add supplements or medicines later as needed. The table below lists selected foods from highest to lowest amounts of tyrosine. (TRYP=L-trypto-phan.)

Selected Foods	Calories	PHE (mg)	TYR (mg)	TRYP (mg)	Fat (grams)	Carbohydrate (grams)	Protein (grams)
Cottage cheese, 1 cup	164	1510	1492	312	2.3	6.2	2.8
Soybeans, boiled, 1 cup	298	1495	1084	416	15.4	17.1	28.6
Chicken breast, 1/2 roasted, w/o skin (100 grams)	193	1146	960	333	7.6	0.0	29.2
Salmon, cooked, 3 oz	127	848	734	243	3.8	0.0	21.7
Herring, cooked, 3 oz	172	764	661	219	9.9	0.0	19.6
Yogurt, low-fat, 8 fl oz	144	650	601	67	3.5	16	11.9
Milk, skim, 8 fl oz	86	403	403	118	0.4	11.9	8.4
Yogurt, whole, 8 fl oz	139	430	398	44	7.4	7.9	10.6
Beans, baked, 1 cup	382	726	392	170	13	54.1	14
Milk, low-fat, 8 fl oz	150	300	388	113	8.2	11.4	8.0
Peanuts, dry-roasted, 1 oz	164	435	365	64	13.9	6.0	6.6
Cheddar cheese, 1 oz	114	372	341	91	9.4	0.4	7.1
Rice, brown, 1 cup	216	260	189	64	1.8	44.8	5.0
Almonds, blanched, 1 oz	174	320	164	48	14.4	5.2	6.0
Egg white (lg)	17	205	137	43	0.0	0.3	3.5
Egg yolk (lg)	59	119	124	33	5.1	0.3	2.8
Strawberry slices, 1 cup	45	27	31	10	0.6	10.5	0.9
Banana, medium	105	43	27	14	0.6	26.7	1.2
Raw apple with skin (med)	81	7.0	6.0	3.0	0.5	21.1	0.3
Cucumber slices, 1/2 cup	7.0	8.0	5.0	2.0	0.1	1.5	0.3

Spirit Pathway
Foods Rich in Tryptophan

L-tryptophan (TRYP) is an amino acid essential to the synthesis of serotonin. The table below ranks selected foods containing trypto-phan from the highest to the lowest amounts. Eat high-tryptophan-containing foods to have enough of this *essential amino acid* in your bloodstream and in your body. Then choose and eat a *high glycemic* food from the next table when you feel the need to have your brain serotonin level boosted a notch or two. Always use food as your first line of remedy. Add supplements and/or other regimens if the food system is not enough for your Spirit Pathway problem.

Selected Foods	Calories	TRYP (mg)	Fat (grams)	Carbohydrate (grams)	Protein (grams)
Chicken breast, 1/2 roasted, w/o skin	193	333	7.6	0.0	29.2
Shrimp, breaded, fried, 3.5 oz	206	256	10.4	9.8	18.2
Turkey breast, roasted, 3.5 oz	126	246	3.5	0.0	22.2
Salmon, pink, cooked, 3 oz	127	243	3.8	0.0	21.7
Lobster, cooked, 3 oz	83	242	0.5	1.1	17.4
Baked beans, 1 cup	382	170	13	54.1	14
Milk, skim, 8 fl oz	86	118	0.4	11.9	8.4
Milk, whole, 8 fl oz	150	113	8.2	11.4	8.0
Sunflower seeds, dry roasted, 1 oz	165	84	14.1	6.8	5.5
Egg, 1 lg, hard/soft boiled	77	76	5.3	0.6	6.3
Potato, baked, with skin	220	73	0.2	51.0	4.7
Spinach, boiled, 1/2 cup	21	36	0.2	3.4	2.7
Broccoli, boiled, 1/2 cup	22	24	0.3	4.0	2.3
Carrots, boiled, 1/2 cup slices	35	23	0.1	8.2	0.9
Banana, 1 medium	105	14	0.6	26.7	1.2
Pumpkin, boiled, mashed, 1/2 cup	24	11	0.1	6.0	0.9

Energy Quotient: Glycemic Index

The rate at which carbohydrates are broken down to simple sugars and enter the bloodstream is called the *glycemic index*. The higher the glycemic index, the faster the food is processed into simpler sugars for rapid absorption and rapid insulin response. From this table you can select foods that have been ranked in order from lowest to highest amount. Use these food selections as indicated by your Pathway regimen and Energy Factor.

LOW-GLYCEMIC FOODS (30% or Less)

Selected Foods	Calories	Fat (grams)	Carbohydrate (grams)	Protein (grams)
Cherries with skin, 10	49	0.7	11.3	0.8
Grapefruit, pink, raw, 1 medium	37	0.1	9.5	0.7
Peach, 1 medium	37	0.1	9.7	0.6
Plum, 1 medium	36	0.4	8.6	0.5
Sausage, smoked, 10 oz	89	7.6	0.7	4.0
Soybeans, boiled, 1 cup	298	15.4	17.1	28.6
Peanuts, dry roasted, 1 oz	164	13.9	6.0	6.6
Red lentils, boiled, 1 cup	231	0.7	39.9	17.9

MODERATE–GLYCEMIC FOODS (30 to 50%)

Selected Foods	Calories	Fat (grams)	Carbohydrate (grams)	Protein (grams)
Golden apple, 1	81	0.5	21.0	0.4
Applesauce, canned, 3.75 oz	72	0.0	17	0.0
Black-eyed peas, boiled, 1 cup	160	0.6	33.5	5.2
Chickpeas, boiled, 1 cup	269	4.3	45	14.5
Milk, low-fat, 8 fl oz	150	8.2	11.4	8.0
Milk, skim, 8 fl oz	86	0.4	11.9	8.4
Sponge cake, 1 piece	188	3.1	4.0	4.0
Sweet potato, 1 cooked	118	0.6	37	2.4
Yogurt, whole, 8 fl oz	139	7.4	7.9	10.6
Yogurt, low-fat, 8 fl oz	144	3.5	16	11.9
Ice cream, 16% high fat, $1/2$ cup	178	12	16.5	2.6
Kidney beans, boiled, 1 cup	225	0.9	40.4	15.4
Tomato soup, 1 cup	160	6.0	22.3	6.1
Apple juice, 6 fl oz	97	0.1	23.7	0.3
Rye bread, whole-grain, 1 slice	66	0.9	12	.1
Pear, 1 medium	98	0.7	25	0.7
Grapes, 1 cup	58	0.3	15.8	0.6
Lima beans, boiled, 1 cup	217	0.7	39.3	14.7

MODERATELY HIGH GLYCEMIC FOODS (50 to 80%)

Selected Foods	Calories	Fat (grams)	Carbohydrate (grams)	Protein (grams)
Banana, 1 large	105	0.6	26.7	1.2
Pumpernickel bread, 1 slice	82	0.8	15.4	2.9
Orange, 1 medium	65	0.3	16	1.3
Roman meal oatmeal rolls, 2	180	3.8	32.2	4.2
Pastry, toasted, 1 oz	195	5.7	35.2	1.9
White bread, 1 slice	64	0.9	11.7	2.0
Corn kernels, $1/2$ cup	89	1.1	20.6	2.7
Beets, boiled, $1/2$ cup slices	26	0.0	5.7	0.9
Spaghetti, cooked, 1 cup	197	0.9	39.7	6.7
All-bran cereal, $1/3$ cup	70	1.0	22	4.0
Orange juice, 6 fl oz	90	0.3	21.4	0.5
Baked beans, 1 cup	382	13	54.1	14.0
Snickers candy bar	277	13.6	36.8	5.8
Potato chips, barbecued, 1 oz	139	9.2	15	2.2
Pinto beans, boiled, $1/2$ cup	235	0.9	43.9	14.0
Green peas, boiled, $1/2$ cup	67	0.2	12.5	4.3

HIGH–GLYCEMIC FOODS (80 to 100%)

Selected Foods	Calories	Fat (grams)	Carbohydrate (grams)	Protein (grams)
Raisins, seedless, ²/₃ cup	302	0.5	79.5	3.4
Apricots, 3 medium	51	0.4	11.8	1.5
Papaya, 1 medium	117	0.4	29.8	1.9
Mango, 1	135	0.6	35.2	1.1
Vanilla ice cream, low-fat, ¹/₂ cup	132	7.3	15.5	2.3
Honey (strained or extracted), 1 T	64	0.0	17.3	0.1
Cornflakes, 1 cup	100	0.1	24.4	2.3
Oat bran, 0.83 oz. bar	110	4.0	16	2.0
Carrot, 1 medium	31	0.1	7.3	0.7
Carrots, boiled, ¹/₂ cup	35	0.1	8.2	0.9
Parsnips, boiled, ¹/₂ cup	63	0.2	15.2	1.0
Corn, boiled, ¹/₂ cup	89	1.1	20.6	2.7
Corn, cream-style, canned, ¹/₂ cup	93	0.5	23.2	2.2
Brown rice, 1 cup	216	1.8	44.8	5.0
Grapenuts cereal, ¹/₄ cup	105	0.1	23.1	3.1
White rice, cooked, ¹/₂ cup	141	2.0	27.4	2.6
Instant mashed potatoes, ¹/₂ cup	130	6.0	17	3.0
Whole wheat bread, 1 slice	61	1.1	11.4	2.4
Lima beans, boiled, 1 cup	217	0.7	39.3	14.7

EXTREMELY HIGH GLYCEMIC FOODS (greater than 100%)

Selected Foods	Calories	Fat (grams)	Carbohydrate (grams)	Protein (grams)
Cornflakes, 1 cup	100	0.1	24.4	2.3
Potato, w/skin, microwaved	156	0.2	36.3	3.3
French bread, 1 slice	81	1.1	14.8	2.7
1 rice cake (puffed)	21	0.0	4.6	0.5

Epilogue
Antiaging Medicine in the Twenty-first Century

What is now proved was once only imagined.
—WILLIAM BLAKE

As I write this at the Sports Medicine & Anti-Aging Medical Group, beside me is a front-page article in the *Los Angeles Times* telegraphing the latest breakthrough in anti-medicine: "Human Chromosome Created Artificially: It May Offer a Way to Cure Inherited Diseases." This startling announcement follows closely on the heels of what has been called the scientific breakthrough of the decade (if not the century): the cloning of a mammal—Dolly, the sheep, to be precise. Together these two developments jump-start the promise of genetic engineering as the ultimate antiaging medical tool. Imagine curing an inherited disease by introducing *therapeutic genetic material* into the patient's cells? Or replacing a faulty organ with one from an animal that has been cloned as a suitable transplant donor for humans? Or ordering from a lab a customized gene package that would prevent the onset of age-related damage and diseases.

Besides gene engineering, a whole array of other antiaging medical tools are on the horizon. Biochemists are working on many new hormones that block fat deposits and suppress appetite. Biotechnologists are developing credit cards that can instantly provide vital statistics for a patient's diagnosis in a medical emergency. Immunotherapists are researching how to adjust white blood T-cells to inhibit or even cure a wide range of diseases, including allergies, asthma, inflammation, and autoimmune diseases. Oral vaccine therapy for dreaded neurodegenerative diseases, such as multiple sclerosis, has already begun.

With these and other antiaging therapies coming soon to a drugstore (or doctor's office) near you, one is reminded of the advertising jingle for a long-distance phone company: "Is this a great time we're living in, or what?" Here's a look at what else is in the works:

Nanotechnology

Called the "manufacturing technology of the twenty-first century," nanotechnology crosses many different fields. It allows us to build a broad range of complex molecular machines, including computers with a molecular architecture. Computer-controlled molecular tools much smaller than a human cell will be built with the accuracy and precision of therapeutic drug molecules. What will these little machines with programmable intelligence do? They will remove obstructions in the circulatory system, kill cancer cells, or take over the function of subcellular oganelles. Just as today we have the artificial heart, in the near future we might have artificial mitochondria, the part of the cell that serves as a power generator.

Equally dramatic, nanotechnology will give us new diagnostic instruments to examine tissue in unprecedented detail. In the classic science fiction film *Fantastic Voyage,* a medical team is reduced to microscopic size and injected into a human body. It's the same concept except for little robots instead of people. Sensors smaller than a cell would give a completely detailed "snapshot" of activities on the cellular, subcellular, molecular, and even atomic levels. There would be no germ too small to detect the probing eye of these sensors.

Cryonics

Cryonics today is all smoke and mirrors, about as close to science as Tomorrowland at Disneyland. But it's not the concept as much as the practice that is in dispute. Cryonics is the deep freezing of human bodies at death, with brain cells still working, to preserve them for eventual revival. The technique achieves the goal of stabilizing human tissue, but the process of freezing at the temperature of liquid nitrogen inflicts a level of cellular damage that cannot be reversed by current technology.

In the twenty-first century, cryonics might be used to stabilize the condition of someone who is seriously injured until treatment becomes available. Or cryonics might be used to preserve human tissue and organs on the death of a person to be used by another. The inability at this time to reverse freezing injury does not mean that a new technology will not overcome the problem. (The computer, after all, was envisioned as early as 1834 by George Babbage and Ada Lovelace.) Current research focuses on nondestructive suspension techniques.

Apoptosis

Neutrophils are specialized cells that maintain the body's immunity by hunting down and killing invading pathogens (viruses, bacteria, and the like). After only one day, these mighty warriors self-destruct, making room for fresh new troops in a process known as *apoptosis,* or programmed cell death. Sometimes this cellular system of self-destruction malfunctions, which can result in uncontrolled cell growth and leukemia. Researchers are developing a variety of cancer drugs to stop or at least fight these good immunity cells that have gone bad.

Cloning

The debut of Dolly, the first cloned mammal, was grist for all sorts of speculation about its effect on aging. First, the bad news. You can't clone your mind. Even if you were so inclined, cloning yourself would simply produce a genetically identical being, an identical twin if you will, but it would not be "you"—the culmination of your memories, experiences, interpersonal relationships, and so forth.

The good news is that cloning will facilitate the breeding of *transgenic* animals whose DNA can be altered so that it will be in tune with the human immune system. Transgenic animals are already used to produce drugs. For example, antithrombin 3, a protein involved in the blood-clotting process, is being produced in the milk of genetically altered goats at a cost far less than biotechnology drugs. Another protein produced by transgenic sheep may be the first effective treatment for cystic fibrosis.

Genetically altered animals could also be valuable sources for replacing human parts. That might sound like shades of *The Island of Dr. Moreau*, but in reality pig valves are routinely used in cardiac surgery. Cloning produces "cleaner" replacement parts with less risk of immune rejection by the human body.

Gene Therapy

Gene therapy, or somatic genetic engineering, is not only a promising new treatment for the ravages of aging, but also offers a whole new paradigm for medicine. Conventional medicine combats disease by using medications, radiation, and surgery to alter the genetic structure of the invading agent and, if all goes well, eliminate it. Gene therapy aims to modify the conditions that make tissue susceptible to disease, essentially correcting the defect by introducing a good genetic material, changing or eliminating the bad material.

Initially, those involved in gene therapy envisioned only the treatment of genetic disorders, but they are now studying a wide range of classically noninherited diseases, including cancer, arthritis, and neurodegenerative disorders, including Lou Gehrig's disease, Parkinson's disease, stroke-induced paralysis and dementias, multiple sclerosis, and other environmentally acquired diseases.

Germline Engineering

As promising as gene therapy is, we most likely will see the results of germline engineering first. The difference is that gene therapy attempts to modify an existing organism while germline engineering focuses on the unborn organism, that is, the unfertilized egg. It is much easier technically to build or insert better artificial chromosomes and other genetic material at the egg stage of a human or animal than correcting a defect after birth. New chromosomes could be developed that could protect future generations from the whole range of diseases and conditions that accelerate aging, including arthritis, osteoporosis, muscle degeneration, memory loss, heart disease, and obesity. In fact, the potential of genetic construction of an ageless human exists with today's technology.

The Human Genome Project, an international effort to map the chemical identity of all 100,000 human genes, will usher in a new age of gene therapy. The project is scheduled for completion by the year 2000, but already it is yielding results. Researchers are focusing not only on genes linked with specific diseases but on aging itself. These are some of the areas being researched:

OSTEOPOROSIS:

Could osteoporosis be a genetic-based disease? A recent paper in *Science* magazine linked brittle bones to a gene associated with an enzyme known as cathepsin K. In healthy human bodies, the enzyme is secreted by a class of cells known as osteoclasts, which are responsible for bone degradation. Osteoclasts are the counterbalance to bond building cells called osteoblasts. By maintaining a careful balance, the two cell types are responsible for normal bone remodeling and skeletal integrity. However, when too much cathepsin K is secreted, bones degrade. Researchers recently announced they had discovered the biostructure of cathepsin K, a major step in the creation of a drug to inhibit or bind the destructive enzyme and possibly arrest the bone-destroying effects of osteoporosis.

OBESITY:

Why is it that some people can eat whatever they want and stay slim, and others just look at a piece of Boston cream pie and feel their fat cells expanding? Researchers at the University of California at Davis, believe the answer lies in a gene that is a blueprint for a protein called UCP2. The researchers found that animals with a high level of UCP2 in their tissues are resistant to weight gain, while those with lower levels gain weight easily. The finding differs from the earlier discovery of leptin, a protein connected with fat accumulation. Studies are now under way to formulate drugs that will tweak the guilty gene to stimulate the secretion of more fat-burning UCP2 in humans.

DIABETES:

The most prevalent form of diabetes is type 2, which affects about 15 million Americans and usually develops in people older than forty, especially those who are overweight. In diabetes, blood sugar rises out of control because the body does not secrete enough insulin or the insulin is not working properly. Scientists have found two genes in a particular strain of type 2 diabetes that sabotage the body's efforts to rein in blood sugar, and this finding may provide an important step to a cure. Surprisingly, the genes seem to have multiple and distinct functions—also regulating activity in the intestine, kidney, and pancreas—adding a new dimension to genetic research.

CANCER:

Oncologists are hoping that a gene called p53, which is implicated in fifty-two types of human cancer, may be the switch that can stop potentially cancerous cells from heading down the wrong path. Ironically, p53 stops tumors before they grow when it functions properly. But when damaged or missing, it is the cause for 60 percent of all cancer deaths, including up to 90 percent of cancer of the cervix, 65 percent of liver cancer, and 50 percent of cancers of the brain and liver. Researchers are now studying ways to jury-rig viruses to carry healthy p53 genes and drugs that mimic the function of p53, turning on genes that halt malignant cell growth or triggering mutant cells to self-destruct. Researchers in Texas have already been successful in shrinking or destroying tumors in lung cancer patients by injecting them with properly functioning p53 genes.

GERMS:

A number of researchers working in the shadow of the vast Human Genome Project are taking a different approach to stopping pathogens, that is, infectious disease-carrying organisms such as viruses and bacteria. Biologists are rapidly deciphering the genetic codes of the germs, offering the possibility of new drugs and vaccines before the Human Genome Project is completed. A major goal of the work is to understand how pathogens evade attack by the body's immune system. "Silico-biologists," who use high-speed computers, are confident that all the major pathogens will be sequenced by the end of the decade.

LIFE SPAN:

The bulk of gene therapy is directed at fixing or replacing defective genes so that the body is no longer susceptible to diseases, age-related or otherwise. But scientists are also looking to discover a genetic way of stopping the aging process itself. A group of researchers in Seattle have identified a human gene that causes Werner's syndrome, a disease whose victims age (and die) prematurely. The discovery has provided researchers with the first look into the complex biochemical processes which produce the debilitating frailties that accompany aging. One in two hundred people carries the defective gene that predisposes humans to cancer and other age-related diseases even though they do not develop Werner's. Another group of researchers in Canada has discovered a set of genes that determine the life span of a nematode, or earthworm, that historically has played an important role in understanding human genetics. By manipulating these genes, which serve as a central biological clock, the biologists were able to extend the worm's life span by 600 percent.

The advances in antiaging medicine, particularly therapy guided by genetic information, open a Pandora's box of questions about life span extension and genetic selection. Should life span technologies and therapies be made available to everyone (including those who can't afford it)? Should certain human embryos be destroyed if it is determined they have genetic defects? And what is a defect—a high risk of breast cancer, short stature, homosexuality? And who decides? If a physician determines his patient has a very high genetic risk of a disease, who has the right to know? The patient's siblings, spouse, children, the physician's HMO, the patient's employer? What if the disease is potentially contagious, should all of society be warned? If everybody lives longer, won't that exacerbate the world's overpopulation problem?

I don't pretend to know the answers to these questions, but here are some thoughts. The human life span is increasing at a fairly dramatic rate even without antiaging therapies. At the turn of the century life expectancy at birth was 47.3 years. In 1994 it was 75.7. To look at it in another way, fewer than 60 percent of women lived to the age of 50 in 1900, while today 95 percent of women can expect to live to at least 50. Antiaging therapies don't promise just to prolong life, they promise to make the quality of life much better.

Chronic ailments such as arthritis, diabetes, and high blood pressure, which affect the elderly in disproportionate numbers, afflict 99 million Americans and cost $470 billion a year in direct health care costs, according to a study recently published in the *Journal of the American Medical Association*. Indirectly, they cost $234 billion in lost productivity. If advanced antiaging therapies can eliminate these illnesses by gene therapy and other treatments, should not at least a portion of that approximately $700 billion in savings be spent on providing antiaging medicine to those who can't afford it?

The discovery of the X-ray tube in 1896 revolutionized medicine, providing for the first time a tool for an objective diagnosis of the interior of the human body and turning what had largely been an art into the beginning of a science. Ethical questions at that time arose as to what is normal and what is abnormal, that is, what needs medical attention and what is a "normal" variation. One hundred years later the development of the sophisticated medical imaging tools known as the ultrasound scan gives parents the opportunity to see their child before it is born. If you believe that the decision to carry a fetus to birth is ultimately the mother's, then should not the same rationale be used when assessing genetic information screened from an egg or sperm?

Many industrialized countries are near or at population growth rates that match replacement levels. In fact, some countries in Europe have birth rates less than replacement levels. Generally speaking, the developed world does not have an overpopulation problem. History indicates that as a nation reaches a certain level of affluence and education, growth rates slow to replacement levels. As information becomes increasingly available through the Internet, satellites and wireless telecommunications, education and, we hope, affluence will reach the undeveloped countries and curtail the current overpopulation crisis.

For the next five to seven years there may be a gap between knowledge and treatment. While the Human Genome Project will finish mapping the 100,000 human genes around 2005, that blueprint for gene therapy will likely sit on the shelf for a few years until new technologies are developed. To date we know how to correct a bad gene in a fertilized egg, but nobody has the foggiest notion how to change or remove a bad gene that is causing heart disease or Alzheimer's in fully developed organisms. On the other hand, this development could come tomorrow. No one in the science community in 1996 would have predicted the breakthrough in genetic cloning that occurred in 1997.

The days of disorder are coming to a close. Our understanding of the causes of aging, already greatly enhanced in the last ten years, are about to take a quantum leap forward. The age-old boundaries already have been crossed, and the path is just ahead to an old age of vigor and vitality. Decades of never-before-experienced opportunities free from disease and disability are in our grasp. The choice is ours if we take a pro-active approach to antiaging today.

See you in the twenty-first century.

Appendix 1:
Antiaging Exercises

With aging the contraction of muscles occurs in three main areas: (1) neck and upper shoulders, and between the shoulder blades, (2) lower back and buttocks, and (3) calves and thighs. This contraction is responsible for much of the lack of mobility that accompanies aging. If these simple stretching, coordination, and strength-building exercises are done daily, they can help ensure a lifetime of fluid movement.

Calf Stretch

- ◆ Objective: Increase the ability to stretch your foot backward.
- ◆ Goal: Prevent calf cramps, and pulls and pain at the arch of your foot (plantar fasciitis).
- ◆ Technique: Find a small step and a rail to hold on to. Let your heels drop off the edge of the step. Second, slightly lift your left leg. Hold the stretch comfortably on the straightened right leg for 30 seconds. Build up to a continuous 60-second stretch. Do the same with the other leg. This stretches out the gastrocnemius muscles that start behind your knee and end at the Achilles tendon. Repeat the exercise, but this time with the right-leg knee bent (your left leg is still slightly lifted). Now you will feel a different stretch that involves the deep muscle of the calf, called the soleus.

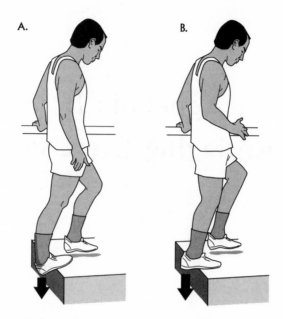

Figure 12—"Calf Stretch"

Hamstring Stretch

◆ Objective: Increase the length of the posterior thigh, called the medial and lateral hamstring muscles.
◆ Goal: Prevent muscle pulls, cramps, and tendinitis. Contracted hamstring muscles contribute to low back pain.
◆ Technique: Put the heel of one foot on a tabletop or chair seat. With your back held straight bend at the waist and feel a pull at the back of your thigh. Increase that pulling sensation by flexing your foot backward. To stretch both the medial and lateral hamstrings, turn your toes out and bend at the waist. Hold for thirty seconds and then turn the toes inward and hold. Return to the starting position and hold another 30 seconds. The total stretch time is 90 seconds for each leg. General rule: Stretching less than 30 seconds does not get to the deep connective tissue fibers within the muscles, which is where the stretch is really needed.

Quadriceps Stretch

◆ Objective: Lengthen the front muscles of your thigh.
◆ Goal: Sitting at a desk or in a car for hours causes these mus-

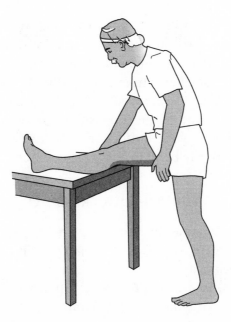

Figure 13—"Hamstring Stretch"

cles to tighten. When you go out for a quick sprint on the weekend, you may feel a stinging, tearing pain at the front of the thigh. The goal is to prevent pulls and cramps.

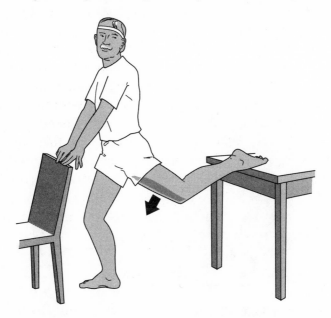

Figure 14—"Quadriceps Stretch"

◆ Technique: Go to your desk or a table, turn your back to it, and lift your foot onto the table or desk, with the heel facing upward. Hold on to the back of a chair placed in front of you. With your back held straight and buttocks pulled in, bend the knee that has all your weight on it. You should feel a stretch across the front of the opposite thigh. If you don't feel a stretch, pull in your buttock muscles more, flatten the back, and increase the bend in the weighted knee.

Gluteal-Buttock Stretch

◆ Objective: Release the lateral hip and buttock muscles.
◆ Goal: Decrease low back pain, lateral hip pain, and bursitis. Prevent sciatica.
◆ Technique: In a sitting position, flatten your back against the wall. With your knees bent, wrap one knee over the other like a pretzel. Place your right hand above your left ankle and grasp it. Take the left hand and place it at the outside of your left knee. Now together pull the left ankle and push the left knee, first toward the right armpit, and hold for 30–45 seconds. Relax. Repeat the same for the other side. Repeat the sequence two more times, increasing the hold to 60 seconds.

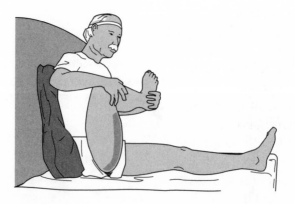

Figure 15—"Gluteal-Buttock Stretch"

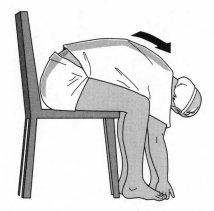

Figure 16—"Spine Stretch"

Spine Stretch

◆ Objective: Lengthen the spinal muscles.
◆ Goal: Relieve low and mid back pain, and prevent injury.
◆ Technique: Sit comfortably in a chair. Bend forward and grab your toes. Feel the stretch of the lower and upper back areas. Stop if you feel dizzy or get a headache. Hold for 10–15 seconds. Repeat as needed.

Neck and Upper Shoulder Stretch

◆ Objective: Increase the range of motion of your neck and upper shoulders.
◆ Goal: Prevent neck spasms, pain, and pulls. To improve neck motion.
◆ Technique 1—Posterior Neck Stretch: Sit up straight in a chair with your chest out and chin in. Turn your head toward the right shoulder and bring your chin downward. Take your left hand and place it under your chair. Put your right hand behind your head and stabilize it. Let go of the chair with your left hand and pull the left arm and shoulder downward. Feel the stretch along the back side of your neck. Remember to let the left shoulder and arm do the pulling. Do not press down on the head with the right hand. Stretch gently for

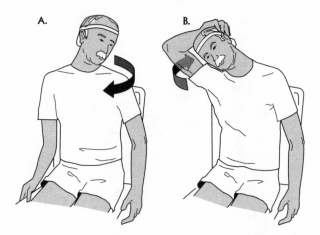

Figure I7—"Neck and Upper Shoulder Stretch"

10–15 seconds. Repeat as needed throughout the day. Do the same for the other side of your neck.

◆ Technique 2—Lateral Neck Stretch: Tilt your head toward the right by aiming your right ear toward the right shoulder. Let the left arm dangle at your side. Place the right hand on the left side of your head. Stabilize the head and stretch the left arm and shoulder downward. You should feel a stretch at the left side of the neck. Remember not to press down on your head with the right hand. The opposite side does the stretch. Hold the stretch for 10–15 seconds. Repeat as needed.

◆ General Rule: All stretches should be done shy of the end range of motion where you feel pain. Always avoid neck extension (bringing the chin up and back) and avoid neck rolls.

Coordination / Balance

◆ Objective: Increase the proprioceptive capacity—the ability to automatically feel where your legs are as you walk or climb stairs or play sports.

◆ Goal: Prevent falls and knee and ankle sprains.

◆ Technique: Walk barefoot, placing one foot in front of the other while looking straight ahead. Touch heel to toe while walking, and try not to sway off to the side. If you tend to drift toward the side, then space your legs farther apart until you can walk without a sway. Repetition is important to train this unconscious system.

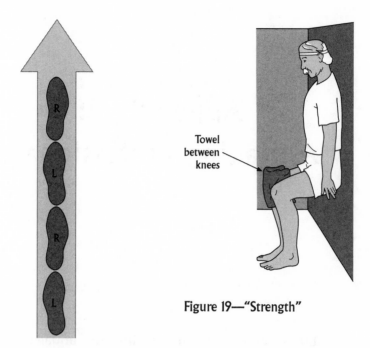

Figure 19—"Strength"

Figure 18—"Coordination / Balance"

Strength

◆ Objective: Strengthen the front thigh muscles (quadriceps).
◆ Goal: Decrease and prevent pain around the kneecap and prevent falls.
◆ Technique—Wall Slides: Put your back against the wall and move your feet away from it until the back is flat (no curves). The back of your head should touch the wall. Put a pillow or rolled-up towel between the knees. Squeeze the pillow or towel tightly while bending the knees and squatting down. Squat to a point of comfort only. Keep squeezing the buttocks and knees together at the same time. The reason is to activate the kneecap-controlling muscle called the vastus medialis obliquous (VMO) and strengthen your front thigh muscles.

Appendix 2:
Antiaging Professionals

Want to find a physician versed in the latest antiaging therapies?
Consult these sources:

Life Extension Foundation
P. O. Box 229120
Hollywood, FL 33022-9120
800-841-5433
E-mail: lef@lef.org
Website: http://www.lef.org
Has a book available of doctors
with an interest in antiaging and
innovative medicine.

Cognitive Enhancement Research
Institute (CERI)
P. O. Box 4029
Menlo Park, CA 94026
415-321-CERI
E-mail: info@ceri.win.net
Website: http://www.ceri.com
Has a list of M.D.'s, D.O.'s, N.D.'s,
and Ph.D.'s who have a special
interest in smart drugs and
antiaging medications.

Los Angeles Gerontology Research
(LAGRG) and Clinical Groups
(LAGCG) include as members
several doctors who are antiaging
specialists. For referrals, contact:
Karlis Ullis, M.D.
E-mail: kullis@ucla.edu
310-829-1990
For meetings contact:
Joe Schulman
Office: 818-362-2358 or
800-933-3322
Fax: 818-364-2647
E-mail: scoles@grg.org
Website: http://www.grg.org
The Research Group has monthly
meetings in Los Angeles, featuring
speakers who are prominent in the
antiaging field.

American College of Advancement
in Medicine
23121 Verdugo Drive, Suite 204
Laguna Hills, CA 92653
949-583-7666, 800-532-3688
Fax: 949-455-9679

American Academy of Anti-Aging
Medicine
1341 W. Fullerton, Suite 111
Chicago, IL 60614
773-528-8500
Fax: 312-528-4333
Website:
http://www.worldhealth.net

International Society of
Orthomolecular Medicine
16 Florence Avenue
Toronto, Ontario, MZN189 Canada
E-mail: centre@orthomed.org
Website:
http://www.orthomed.org

Appendix 3:
Antiaging Supplement Suppliers

Can't find a particular supplement in your local area? These manufacturers, distributors, and retailers specialize in vitamins, nutrients, herbs and other antiaging products.

Allergy Research Group
P.O. Box 55907
Hayward, CA 94544
800-545-9960
Fax: 510-487-8682

Amni Advanced Medical
Nutrition, Inc.
2247 National Avenue
Hayward, CA 94545 or
P.O. Box 5012
Hayward, CA 94540-5012
800-437-8888

ASTAK
29949 S.R. 54 West
Wesley Chapel, FL 33543
813-973-7902
Fax: 813-973-7002
ASTAK distributes the liquid

DHEA product developed by
Discovery Experimental &
Development, Inc.

Beyond A Century
HC 76, Box 200
Greenville, ME 04441
800-777-1324
Fax: 207-695-2492

CFIDS Buyers Club &
Fibromyalgia Health Resource
1187 Coast Village Road, #1-280
Santa Barbara, CA 93108
800-366-6056
Fax: 805-965-0042
Website:
http://www.prohealthdirect.com

Ecological Formulas
1061-B Shary Circle
Concord, CA 94518
800-888-4585
Fax: 510-676-9231

Free Life International
333 Quarry Rd.
Milford, CT 06450
203-882-7250
800-882-7240 (orders only)
Supplier of Earl Mindell's line of
supplements.

Gero Vita International
32 Larson St.
Markham, Ontario
L3R 1B6 Canada
800-694-8366

Health Center for Better Living
1414 Rosemary Lane
Naples, FL 33942-4283
800-544-4225
Fax: 941-643-6335

HealthCom International, Inc.
5800 Soundview Dr.
Gig Harbor, WA 98335
800-843-9660, 800-851-3943
Fax: 253-851-9749

Herbs of Grace
Division of School of Natural
Medicine
P. O. Box 7369
Boulder, CO 80306-7369
303-443-4882
Fax: 303-443-8276

Jarrow Formulas, Inc.
1824 S. Robertson Blvd.

Los Angeles, CA 90035-4317
800-726-0886; 310-204-6936
Fax: 310-204-2520

L & H Vitamins
32-33 47th Ave.
Long Island City, NY 11101
800-221-1152
Fax: 718-361-1437

Life Enhancement Products
P.O. Box 751390
Petaluma, CA 94975
800-543-3873
Fax: 707-769-8016

Life Extension Foundation
P. O. Box 229120
Hollywood, FL 33022
800-544-4440
Fax: 954-761-9199

LifeLink, A Delano Company
P. O. Box 1299
Grover Beach, CA 93483
805-473-1389; 888-4-DELANO
Fax: 805-473-2803
Website:
http://www.lifelinknet.com

Life Services Supplements, Inc.
3535 Highway 66, Bldg. 2
Neptune, NJ 07753
800-542-3230
Fax: 732-922-5329
Website:
http://www.lifeservices.com
E-mail: email@lifeservices.com

Metagenics Inc.
971 Calle Negocio
San Clemente, CA 92673

800-692-9400
Fax: 714-366-2859

Nu BioLogics, Inc.
30 W. 100 Butterfield Road
Warrenville, IL 60555-1512
800-3332-3130; 630-393-7500
Fax: 630-393-7590

Nutrition Plus
4747 E. Elliot Road, Suite 29
Phoenix, AZ 85044
800-241-9236
Fax: 303-872-3862

Olympia Nutrition
3579 Highway 50 East, Suite 220
Carson City, NV 89701
888-366-9909
Fax: 619-270-9095
E-mail: olympia@smart-drugs.com
Website:
http://www.smart-drugs.com

Peggy's Health Center
151 First Street
Los Altos, CA 94022
800-862-9191
Fax: 650-941-9512
Website:
http://www.inetbiz.com/peggys

Peruvian Rainforest Botanicals
800-742-2529
Fax: 561-745-3017
Website:
http://www.nutrimedi.com

Pharmacognosy-22
1945 East Ridge Road,
Suite 5288

Rochester, NY 14622
1-800-5NEURON (563-8766)

Smart Basics
1626 Union St.
San Francisco, CA 94123
800-878-6520; 415-749-3990
Website:
http://www.smartbasic.com
E-mail: orders@smartbasic.com

Source Naturals
23 Janis Way
Scotts Valley, CA 95066
831-438-1144
Fax: 831-438-7410

Tyler Encapsulations
2204 N.W. Birdsdale
Gresham, OR 97030
800-869-9705; 503-661-5401
Fax: 503-666-4913

Vitamin Express
1428 Irving Street
San Francisco, CA 94122
415-564-8160
Fax: 800-218-7900
Website:
http://www.vitaminexpress.com
A health food store with an
extensive number of items. Also
publishes a newsletter.

Vitamin Research Products
3579 Highway 50 East
Carson City, NV 89701
800-VRP-24HR
E-mail: mail@vrp.com

The Vitamin Shop
4700 Westside Avenue
North Bergen, NJ 07047
800-223-1216

Wellness Health &
Pharmaceuticals
2800 South 18th Street
Birmingham, AL 35209
800-227-2627
Fax: 1-800-369-0302

NOTE: There has been no objective evaluation of the suppliers listed regarding their products or services. This is a partial guide for your antiaging supplement needs and does not constitute an endorsement of any kind.

Appendix 4:
Diagnostic Laboratories

The following labs provide at-home antiaging tests, which are useful in determining your biological age and the progress of your antiaging regimen. None requires a doctor's prescription, but some of the test results may need to be interpreted by a doctor or other knowledgeable health care professional.

Aeron Lifecycles
1933 Davis St., Suite 310
San Leandro, CA 94577
800-631-7900
Fax: 510-729-0383
Website:
http://www.aeron@aeron.com

Diagnos-Techs, Inc., Clinical
Research and Laboratory
6620 South 192nd Pl., J-104
Kent, WA 98032
800-878-3787
Fax: 425-251-0637
E-mail: diagnos@diagnostechs.com

Great Smokies Diagnostic
Laboratory
63 Zillicoa St.
Asheville, NC 28801
704-253-0621
Fax: 828-253-1127

Genox Corporation
1414 Key Highway
Baltimore, MD 21230
410-347-7616
Fax: 410-347-7617
Website: http://www.genox.com
E-mail: info@genox.com

Immunosciences Lab., Inc.
8730 Wilshire Blvd., Suite 305
Beverly Hills, CA 90211
310-657-1077, 800-950-4686
Fax: 310-657-1053

LXN Corporation
5830 Oberlin Drive
San Diego, CA [no zip code listed]
1-888-LXN-TEST
Website: http://www.lxncorp.com

MetaMetrix, Inc.
5000 Peachtree Industrial Blvd.,
Suite 110
Norcross, GA 30071
800-221-4640
770-446-5483
Fax: 771-441-2237

Meridian Valley Clinical
Laboratory
515 West Harrison, #9
Kent, WA 98032
253-859-8700

Pantox Laboratories
4622 Santa Fe St.
San Diego, CA 92109
619-272-3885, 800-PANTOX6
(726-8696)

Appendix 5:
Consumer's Guide
to Hormone Replacement
DHEA, Melatonin, and Pregnenolone

DHEA, melatonin, and pregnenolone, naturally occurring hormones in the body, are available as over-the-counter supplements. Found in the brain, they are called *neuro*hormones because they affect hormonal systems of the brain and body.

DHEA and pregnenolone are precursor hormones—chemical foundations—for the sex hormone and others. By taking these precursors you are letting your body decide what other hormones to make from them. In other words, their effect is unpredictable. For example, DHEA may increase testosterone levels in some men, but in others it might increase estrogen levels.

Melatonin has a regulatory effect on our night–day hormone secretion patterns. All three hormones should be taken with a degree of caution and with an awareness of possible adverse or unintended side effects. Take a "hormone holiday" periodically; that is, stop taking them. The body must rebalance itself after taking these hormones. Their effects can last up to several days after you stop. After the "holiday" readjustment period, a new therapeutic cycle can be started.

Consult with a medical doctor if you currently are on a hormone replacement program and before exceeding the amounts and frequency of the doses recommended below.

Maximum Dosages

- ◆ DHEA 25 mg
- ◆ Pregnenolone 15 mg
- ◆ Melatonin 3 mg

Consult with a health practitioner as to the frequency and duration of your hormone holidays. A reasonable approach is to stop using the hormones a day or two per week or up to a week or two per month.

Men: Ages forty to fifty

Melatonin: 0.1 to 0.5 mg once or twice per week before bedtime, as needed for sleep or for Pathway antiaging effects.

Pregnenolone: 1–5 mg in the morning every other day with frequent hormone holidays.

DHEA: 5–10 mg every other day with frequent hormone holidays to avoid suppressing your natural testosterone production.

Caution: The combined total daily dose of pregnenolone and DHEA is not to exceed 15 mg.

Men: Ages fifty to sixty-five

Melatonin: 0.3 to 2 mg one to three times a week before bedtime as needed for sleep or for Pathway antiaging effects.

Pregnenolone: 5–10 mg in the morning every other day with frequent hormone holidays.

DHEA: 5–20 mg every other day with frequent hormone holidays, to avoid suppressing your natural testosterone production, or for the possible conversion of DHEA to estrogen.

Caution: The combined total daily dose of pregnenolone and DHEA is not to exceed 30 mg.

Men: Ages sixty-five and older

Melatonin: 0.3 to 3 mg one to three times per week at bedtime as needed for sleep. Consider 0.3 to 0.5 mg nightly for chronic insomnia or for Pathway antiaging effects.

Pregnenolone: 5–15 mg in the morning every other day with occasional hormone holidays.

DHEA: 10–25 mg every other day with occasional hormone holidays. High doses and excessive use can have a negative impact on the prostate gland or cause a rise in estrogen levels.

Caution: The combined total daily dose of pregnenolone and DHEA is not to exceed 40 mg.

Premenopausal Women: Ages forty to about fifty

Melatonin: 0.1 to 0.5 mg once or twice a week before bedtime, as needed for sleep or for Pathway antiaging effects. Keep the doses very low or don't use at all if contemplating pregnancy; melatonin in larger doses is being investigated as a contraceptive.

Pregnenolone: 1–5 mg every other day with frequent hormone holidays.

DHEA: 5–10 mg every other day with frequent hormone holidays.

Caution: The combined daily dose of pregnenolone and DHEA is not to exceed 15 mg.

Postmenopausal Women: Ages fifty to sixty-five

Melatonin: 0.2 to 2 mg once or twice a week before bedtime, as needed for sleep or for Pathway antiaging effects.

Pregnenolone: 5–10 mg every other day with occasional hormone holidays.

DHEA: 5–15 mg every other day with occasional hormone holidays.

Caution: The combined daily dose of pregnenolone and DHEA is not to exceed 25 mg.

Women: Ages sixty-five and over

Melatonin: 0.3 to 3 mg one to three times per week before bedtime, as needed for sleep. Consider taking 0.1 to 0.5 mg nightly for chronic insomnia or for Pathway antiaging effects.

Pregnenolone: 5–15 mg every other day with occasional hormone holidays.

DHEA: 5–20 mg every other day with occasional hormone holidays.

Caution: The combined daily dose of pregnenolone and DHEA is not to exceed 35 mg.

Source: Conceptual framework adapted from *The New Memory Boosters: Natural Supplements That Enhance Your Mind, Memory, and Mood* by Ray Sahelian, M.D.

Bibliography

Chapter 1: Why We Age

Finch, Galeb, E. *Longevity, Senescence, and the Genome*. Chicago: University of Chicago Press, 1990.

Macieira-Coelho, Alvaro, ed. *Molecular Basis of Aging*. Boca Raton, FL: CRC Press, Inc., 1995.

Pierpaoli, W.; Regelson, W.; and Fabris, N. (eds.). "The Aging Clock: The Pineal Gland and Other Pacemakers in the Progression of Aging and Carcinogenesis," *Annals of the New York Academy of Sciences* 719 (1994).

Ricklefs, Robert E., and Finch, Caleb E. *Aging: A Natural History*. New York: Scientific American Library, 1995.

Wright, Janice C., Ph.D., and Weinstein, Michael, Ph.D. "Gains in Life Expectancy from Medical Intervention—Standardizing Data on Outcomes," *The New England Journal of Medicine* 339 (Aug. 6, 1998), 380–86.

Zs-Nagy, Imre. *The Membrane Hypothesis of Aging*. Boca Raton, FL: CRC Press, 1994.

Chapter 2: How We Age

Dilman, Vladimir M., M.D., and Ward, Dean, M.D. *The Neuroendocrine Theory of Aging and Degenerative Disease*. Pensacola, FL: The Center for Bio-Gerontology, 1992.

Harman, Denham. "Aging and Disease: Extending Functional Life Span, Pharmacological Intervention in Aging and Age-Associated Disorders," *Annals of the New York Academy of Sciences* 786 (1996), 71–92.

———. "Role of Antioxidant Nutrients in Aging: Overview," *Journal of Age*.

International Association of Biomedical Gerontology, Inc.; American College of Clinical Gerontology, Inc.; American Aging Association, Inc., 8(no. 2) (Apr. 1995): 51–62.

Hayflick, Leonard. *How and Why We Age*. New York: Ballantine Books, 1990.

Penzes, L.; Fischer, H.D.; and Noble, R.C. "Some Aspects on the Relationship Between Lipids, Neurotransmitters, and Aging," *Zeitschrift für Gerontologie* 26(2): 65–69.

Rose, Michael R., *Evolutionary Biology of Aging*. New York: Oxford University Press, 1991.

Shigenega, Mark K.; Hagen, Tory M.; and Ames, Bruce N. "Oxidative Damage and Mitochondrial Decay in Aging," *National Academy of Science, USA* 91 (Nov. 1994): 1077–78.

Walford, Roy L., and Walford, Lisa. *The Anti-Aging Plan, Strategies and Recipes for Extending Your Healthy Years*. New York: Four Walls Eight Windows, 1994.

Wickelgren, Ingrid. "The Aging Brain: For the Cortex, Neuron Loss May Be Less Than Thought," *Science* 273 (July 5, 1996): 48–50.

Chapter 3: Antiaging Medicine: History and Theories

Fossel, Michael, M.D. *Reversing Human Aging*. New York: William Morrow, 1996.

Georgakas, Dan. *The Methuselah Factors: Learning from the World's Longest Living People*. Chicago, Illinois: Academy Chicago Publishers, 1995.

Jazwinkski, S. Michal. "Longevity, Genes, and Aging," *Science* 273 (July 5, 1996): 54–58.

Joseph, J. A. et al., "Increased Sensitivity to Oxidative Stress and the Loss of Muscarinic Receptor Responsiveness in Senescence," *Annals of the New York Academy of Sciences*. New York: New York Academy of Sciences (1995): 112–18.

Odawara, Masato. "Involvement of Mitochondrial Gene Abnormalities in the Pathogenesis of Diabetes Mellitus," *Annals of the New York Academy of Sciences*. New York: New York Academy of Sciences, 1996.

Moore, Thomas J. *Life Span: Who Lives Longer and Why*. New York: Simon and Schuster, 1993.

Olshansky, S. Jay; Carnes, Bruce A.; and Cassel, Christine A. "The Aging of the Human Species," *Scientific American* (Apr. 1993): 46–52.

Shigenega, Mark K.; Hagen, Tory M.; and Ames, Bruce N. "Oxidative Damage and Mitochondrial Decay in Aging," *Proceedings of the National Academy of Science, USA* (Nov. 1994): 10771–78.

Sohal, Rajindar S., and Weindruch, Richard. "Oxidative Stress, Caloric Restriction, and Aging," *Science* 273 (July 5, 1996): 59–63.

Weindruch, Richard. "Caloric Restriction and Aging," *Scientific American* 274(1) (Jan. 1996): 46–52.

Zs-Nagy, Imre. *The Membrane Hypothesis of Aging.* Boca Raton, FL: CRC Press, 1994.

Chapter 4: The Critical Point and the Theory of Human Thermodynamics

Arner, P. "Impact of Exercise on Adipose Tissue Metabolism in Humans," *International Journal of Obesity and Related Metabolic Disorders* 19 Suppl. 4 (Oct. 1995): S18–21.

Brass, E. P., and Hiatt, W.R. "Carnitine Metabolism During Exercise," *Life Sciences* 54, no. 19 (1994): 1383–93.

Di Pasquale, Mauro G. (ed.). "Maximizing Athletic Performance Without Drugs," *Drugs in Sports* 1, no. 2 (May 1992): 10–12.

———. *The Anabolic Diet,* Toronto, Canada: Optimum Training Systems, 1995.

———. *Body Building Supplement Review,* Toronto, Canada. Optimum Training Systems,1995.

Ghigo, E., et al. "Effectiveness of 15-Day Treatment with Growth-Hormone-Releasing Hormone Alone or Combined with Different Doses of Arginine on the Reduced Somatotrope Responsiveness to the Neurohormone in Normal Aging," *European Journal of Endocrinology* 132 (1995): 32–36.

Graham, T. E., and Spriet, L. L. "Metabolic, Catecholamine, and Exercise Performance Responses to Various Doses of Caffeine," *Journal of Applied Physiology* 78, no. 3 (Mar. 1995): 867–74.

Hakkinen, K. "Neuromuscular and Hormonal Adaptations During Strength and Power Training: A Review," *Journal of Sports Medicine and Physical Fitness* 29, no. 1 (Mar. 1989): 9–26.

Hood, D. A., and Terjung, R. L., "Amino Acid Metabolism During Exercise and Following Endurance Training," *Sports Medicine* 9, no. 1 (Jan. 1990): 23–35.

Klein, S. et al. "Effect of Endurance Training on Glycerol Kinetics During Strenuous Exercise in Humans," *Metabolism: Clinical and Experimental* 45, no. 3 (Mar. 1996): 357–61.

Matthews, Dwight E., and Battezzati, Alberto, M.D. "Regulation of Protein Metabolism During Stress," *Current Opinion in General Surgery* (1993): 72–77.

Millward, D.J. et al. "Clinical Aspects of Protein and Energy Metabolism: Whole-Body Protein and Amino Acid Turnover in Man: What Can We Measure with Confidence?" *Proceedings of the Nutrition Society* 50 (1991): 197–216.

Pestell, R. G.; Hurley, D. M.; and Vandongen, R. "Biochemical and Hormonal Changes During a 1000 km Ultramarathon," *Clinical and Experimental Pharmacology and Physiology* 16, no. 5 (May 1989): 353–61.

Stefanick, Marcia L., Ph.D.; Mackey, Sally, M.S., R.D.; Sheehan, Mary, M.S.; Ellsworth, Nancy; Haskell, William L., Ph.D., and Wood, Peter D., D.Sc., Ph.D. "Effects of Diet and Exercise in Men and Postmenopausal Women with Low Levels of HDL Cholesterol and High Levels of LDL Cholesterol," *The New England Journal of Medicine* 339 (July 2, 1998): 12–20.

Tsai, L., et al. "Basal Concentrations of Anabolic and Catabolic Hormones in Relation to Endurance Exercise After Short-Term Changes in Diet," *European Journal of Applied Physiology and Occupational Physiology* 66, no. 4 (1993): 304–8.

Urhausen, A.; Holger, G.; and Kindermann, W. "Blood Hormones as Markers of Training Stress and Overtraining," *Sports Medicine* 20 (Oct. 1995): 251–76.

Chapter 5: The Magic Bullet: Hormonal Harmony and the Growth Hormone Family

Borer, K. T. "Neurohumoral Mediation of Exercise-Induced Growth," *Medicine and Science in Sports and Exercise* 26, no. 6 (June 1994): 741–54.

Conn, Michael, and Bowers, Cyril Y. "A New Receptor for Growth Hormone-Release Peptide," *Science* 273 (Aug. 16, 1996): 923.

Copinschi, G. et al. "Effects of a 7-Day Treatment with a Novel, Orally Active, Growth Hormone (GH) Secretagogue, MK-677, on 24-Hour GH Profiles, Insulin-like Growth Factor I, and Adrenocortical Function in Normal Young Men," *Journal of Clinical Endocrinology and Metabolism* 81, no. 8 (1996): 2776.

Corpas, E., et al. "Oral Arginine-Lysine Does Not Increase Growth Hormone or Insulin-like Growth Factor I in Old Men," *Journal of Gerontology: Medical Sciences* 48, no. 4 (1993): 128–33.

De Boer, H.; Blok, G. J.; and Van der Veen, E. A. "Clinical Aspects of Growth Hormone Deficiency in Adults," *Endocrine Reviews* 16, no. 1 (1995): 63–88.

Di Pasquale, Mauro, M.D. "Dietary Protein: The Anabolic Edge," *Anabolic Research Review* 1, no. 3 (1996): 1–3.

———. "High-Tech Supplementation," *Anabolic Research Review* 1, no. 5 (1996): 5–10.

———. "Increasing Endogenous Testosterone," *Drugs in Sports* 2, no. 1 (Sept. 1993): 11–15.

Di Pasquale, Mauro, M.D., and Thoburn, Robert W. "ATP and the Muscle Hypertropic Response to Exercise," *Anabolic Research Review* 1(1) 1995: 9–12.

Hargreaves, Mark. *Exercise Metabolism.* Champaign, IL: Human Kinetics Publishers, 1995.

Harvey, S.; Scanes, C.; and Daughaday, W. *Growth Hormone.* Boca Raton, FL: CRC Press, 1995.

Howard, A. D.; Feighner, S. D.; and Cully, D. F. "Receptor in Pituitary and Hypothalamus That Functions in Growth Hormone Release," *Science* 273 (Aug. 16, 1996): 974–77.

Keim, N. L., et al. "Moderate Diet Restriction Alters the Substrate and Hormone Response to Exercise," *Medicine and Science in Sports and Exercise* 26, no. 5 (May 1994): 599–604.

Klatz, Ronald, and Kahn, Carol. *Grow Young with HGH: The Amazing Medically Proven Plan to Reverse Aging*. New York: HarperCollins, 1997.

Lamb, David R., and Williams, Melvin H. *Perspectives in Exercise Science and Sports Medicine: Ergogenics Enhancement of Performance in Exercise and Sport*. Carmel, Indiana: Cooper Publishing Group, 1991.

Meeusen, R., and De Meirleir K. "Exercise and Brain Neurotransmission," *Sports Medicine* 20, no. 3 (Sept. 1995): 160–88.

Melmed, Shlomo. *The Pituitary*. England: Blackwell Science, 1995.

Phillips, Bill. *1996 Supplement Review*. Golden,CO: Mile High Publishing, 1995.

Powrie, Jake; Weissberger, Andrew; and Sonksen, Peter. "Growth Hormone Replacement Therapy for Growth-Hormone-Deficient Adults," *Drugs* 49, no. 5 (1995): 656–63.

Saenger, Paul. "Editorial: Oral Growth Hormone Secretagogues—Better Than Alice in Wonderland's Growth Elixir?" *Journal of Clinical Endocrinology and Metabolism* 81, no. 8 (1996): 2773–75.

Sonksen, P. H., and Howard, B. V., "GH: Aging Abstracts," *Endocrinology and Metabolism* 4, Suppl. A, London: Bailliere Tindall Limited (Jan. 1997).

Souba, Wiley W., M.D. "Drug Therapy: Nutritional Support," *The New England Journal of Medicine* 336, no. 1 (Jan. 2, 1997): 41–46, 69–70.

Strasburger, C. J.; Feldmeier, H.; and Nass, R. "Growth Hormone Deficiency in Adulthood," *Topical Endocrinology*, Suppl. 1, E. Lilly Corp. (Mar. 1996) 2–16.

Thoburn, Robert W. "Supplement Update," *Anabolic Research Review* 1, no. 3 (1995): 3–5.

———. "Anabolics Research: Antiglucocorticoid Activity of RU486," *Anabolic Research Review* 1, no. 3 (1995): 6.

Chapter 6: The Four Dimensions of Aging

Besser, G. Michael, and Thorner, Michael O. *Clinical Endocrinology*, 2nd ed., Mosby-Wolfe, 1994.

Birkmayer, W., and Riederer P. *Understanding the Neurotransmitters: Key to the Workings of the Brain*. New York: Springer-Verlag, 1986.

Gilbert, Christine. "Optimal Physical Performance in Athletes: Key Roles of Dopamine in a Specific Neurotransmitter/Hormonal Mechanism," *Mechanisms of Ageing and Development* 84 (1995): 83–102.

Harris, Raymond, M.D., and Harris, Sara. *Physical Activity, Aging and Sports: Scientific and Medical Research*, vol. 1. Albany, New York: Center for the Study of Aging, 1989.

Harris, Sara; Heikkinen, Eino, M.D.; Harris, Willard, M.D. *Physical Activity, Aging and Sports: Toward Healthy Aging—International Perspectives. Part 2: Psychology, Motivation and Programs*, vol. 4, Albany, New York: Center for the Study of Aging, 1995.

Meeusen, Romain, and De Meirleir, Kenny. "Exercise and Brain Neuro-transmission," *Sports Medicine* 20, no. 3 (1995): 160–88.

Nygren, Jonas et al. "Disturbed Anabolic Hormonal Patterns in Burned Patients: The Relation to Glucagon," *Clinical Endocrinology* 43 (1995): 491–500.

Pierpaoli, Walter, M.D.; Regelson, William, M.D.; and Colman, Carol. *The Melatonin Miracle: Nature's Age-Reversing, Disease-Fighting, Sex-Enhancing Hormone.* New York: Simon and Schuster, 1995.

Reid, David C. *Sports Injury Assessment and Rehabilitation.* New York: Churchill Livingstone, Inc., 1992.

Roth, G. S. "Changes in Tissue Responsiveness to Hormones and Neuro-transmitters During Aging," *Experimental Gerontology* 30, nos. 3–4 (May–Aug. 1995): 361–68.

Sahelian, Ray, M.D., *Melatonin: Nature's Sleeping Pill.* Marina del Rey, CA: Be Happier Press, 1995.

Zaman, Z. et al. "Plasma Concentrations of Vitamins A and E and Carotenoids in Alzheimer's Disease," *Age And Ageing* 21, no. 2 (Mar. 1992): 91–94.

Chapter 7: Your Mind-Body-Spirit Quotient

Bland, Jeffrey, and Benum, Sara. *The 20-Day Rejuvenation Diet Program.* New Canaan, CT: Keats Publishing, 1997.

Fratiglioni, L. "Epidemiology of Alzheimer's Disease and Current Possibilities for Prevention," *Acta Neurologica Scandinavica* 165 (1996): 33–40.

Goldfinger, Stephen E., M.D.; Garnett, Leah R.; and Gillyatt, Peta. "Vitamins and Minerals," Harvard Health Letter (Sept. 1995): 60–51.

Lowe, Daniel K., et al. "Safety of Glutamine-Enriched Parenteral Nutrient Solutions in Humans," *American Journal of Clinical Nutrition* 52 (1990): 1101–6.

Malinow, Manuel R., M.D.; Duell, Paul B., M.D.; Hess, David L., Ph.D.; Anderson, Peter H., Ph.D.; Kruger, Warren D., M.D.; Phillipson, Beverley E., M.D.; Gluckman, Robert A., M.D.; Block, Peter C., M.D.; and Upson, Barbara M., B.S., "Reduction of Plasma Homocystine Levels by Breakfast Cereal Fortified with Folic Acid in Patients with Coronary Heart Disease," *The New England Journal of Medicine,* 338 (April 19, 1998), 1009–15.

Rozencwaig, Roman, M.D., and Walji, Hasnain. *The Melatonin and Aging Sourcebook.* Prescott, AZ: Hohm Press, 1997.

Schulkin, Jay. *Hormonally Induced Changes in Mind and Brain.* San Diego, CA: Academic Press, 1993.

Sinatra, Stephen T., M.D. *Optimum Health.* Gatlinburg, TN: Lincoln-Bradley Publishing Group, 1996.

Sojka, J. E., and Weaver, C. M. "Magnesium Supplementation and Osteoporosis," *Nutrition Reviews* 53, no. 3 (1992): 71–80.

Thomas, Melissa K., Ph.D.; Loyd-Jones, Donald M., M.D.; Thadhani, Ravi I., M.D., M.O.H.; Shaw, Albert C., M.D., Ph.D.; Deraska, Donald J.,

M.D.; Kitch, Barrett T., M.D.; Vamvakas, Eleftherios C., M.D., Ph.D.; Dick, Ian M., M.Sc.; Prince, Richard L., M.D., and Finkelstein, Joel. S., M.D., "Hypovitaminosis D in Medical Inpatients," *The New England Journal of Medicine* 338 (Mar. 19, 1998): 777–83.

Timiras, Paola S.; Quay, Wilbur D.; and Vernadakis, Antonia. *Hormones and Aging.* Boca Raton, FL: CRC Press, 1995.

Chapter 8: Mind Pathway

Alcar, Mezzina, et al. "Acetyl L-Carnitine: Natural Substance That Can Be Used to Treat Neurologic Diseases (Idiopathic Facial Paralysis: New Therapeutic Prospects)," *International Journal, Pharmacology Research* 12, nos. 5–6 (1992): 299–304.

Blusztajn, J. K. "Alzheimer's Disease: Prevention, Models, and Diagnostic Tools," *Neurobiology of Aging,* Suppl. 15, no. 2 (1994): S37–39.

Breitner, J. C. "The Role of Anti-inflammatory Drugs in the Prevention and Treatment of Alzheimer's Disease," *Annual Review of Medicine* 47 (1996): 401–11.

Brown, A. S., and Gershon S. "Dopamine and Depression," *Journal of Neural Transmission* 91 (1993): 75–109.

Cummings, Jeffrey and Benson, Frank D. *Dementia: A Clinical Approach,* Boston: Butterworth-Heinemann, 1992.

Fratiglioni, L. "Epidemiology of Alzheimer's Disease and Current Possibilities for Prevention," *Acta Neurologica Scandinavica,* Suppl. 165 (1996): 33–40.

Harman, Denham. "A Hypothesis on the Pathogenesis of Alzheimer's Disease," *Annals of the New York Academy of Sciences.* New York: New York Academy of Sciences, 1995.

Maurizi, C. P. "The Mystery of Alzheimer's Disease and Its Prevention by Melatonin," *Medical Hypotheses* 45, no. 4 (Oct. 1995): 339–40.

Timiras, Paola S. *Physiological Basis of Aging and Geriatrics,* 2nd ed. Boca Raton, FL: CRC Press, 1994.

Zeisel, Steven H., and Blusztajn, Jan K. "Choline and Human Nutrition," *Annual Review Nutrition* 14 (1994): 269–96.

Chapter 9: Body Pathway

Anderson, James W., and Breecher, Maury M. *Dr. Anderson's Antioxidant, Antiaging Health Program,* New York: Carroll & Graf, 1996.

Bennett, David A., et al. "Prevalence of Parkinsonian Signs and Associated Mortality in a Community Population of Older People," *New England Journal of Medicine* 334, no. 2: 71–76.

Dow, Alastair. *Deprenyl, the Anti-Aging Drug,* Delavan, WI: Hallberg Publishing Corporation, 1993.

Fernstrom, John D. "Stress and Monoamine Neurons in the Brain," *Food Components to Enhance Performance,* Washington, D.C.: National Academy Press (1994): 161–67.

Gilbert C. "Optimal Physical Performance in Athletes: Key Roles of

Dopamine in a Specific Neurotransmitter/Hormonal Mechanism," *Mechanisms of Ageing and Development* 84, no. 2 (Oct. 13, 1995): 83–102.

Goetz, C. G., Tanner, C. M., and Klawans, H. L. "Dopaminergic Agonists in the Treatment of Advanced Parkinson's Disease," *The Comprehensive Management of Parkinson's Disease*, Costa Mesa, CA: PMA Publishing (1988): 159–69.

Ivy, John L. *Food Components to Enhance Performance*, Washington, DC: National Academy Press (1994): 233–460.

Lehnert, Hendrik, and Wurtman, Richard J. "Amino Acid Control of Neurotransmitter Synthesis and Release: Physiological and Clinical Implications," *Psychother Psychosom* 60 (1993): 18–32.

Marsden, C.D. "The Drug Therapy of Early Parkinson's Disease," *The Comprehensive Management of Parkinson's Disease*. Costa Mesa, CA: PMA Publishing (1988): 79–87.

Marx, Jean. "Neurodegenerative Disease: Searching for Drugs That Combat Alzheimer's," *Science* 273 (July 5, 1996): 50–53.

Olanow, C. W.; Jenner, P.; and Youdim, M. *Neurodegeneration and Neuroprotection in Parkinson's Disease*. London: Academic Press, 1996.

Packer, L.; Hiramatsu, M.; and Yoshikawa, T. *Free Radicals in Brain Physiology and Disorders*. San Diego, CA: Academic Press, 1996.

Roth, George S., and Joseph, James A. "Cellular and Molecular Mechanisms of Impaired Dopaminergic Function During Aging," *Annals of the New York Academy of Sciences*. New York: New York Academy of Sciences, 1996.

Chapter 10: Spirit Pathway

Cangiano, C., et al. "Eating Behavior and Adherence to Dietary Prescriptions in Obese Adult Subjects Treated with 5-Hydroxytryptophan," *American Journal of Clinical Nutrition* 56 (1992): 863–67.

Davis, J. M., et al. "Effects of Carbohydrate Feedings on Plasma Free Tryptophan and Branched-Chain Amino Acids During Prolonged Cycling," *European Journal of Applied Physiology and Occupational Physiology* 65, no. 6 (1992): 513–19.

Holden, R. J. "Schizophrenia, Suicide and the Serotonin Story," *Medical Hypotheses* 44 (1995): 379–91.

Lehnert, H., and Wurtman, R. J. "Amino Acid Control of Neurotransmitter Synthesis and Release: Physiological and Clinical Implications," *Psychotherapy and Psychosomatics* 60, no. 1 (1993): 18–32.

Mullen, B. J., and Martin, R. J. "The Effect of Dietary Fat on Diet Selection May Involve Central Serotonin," *American Journal of Physiology* 263, no. 3, part 2 (Sept. 1992): R559–63.

Pijl, H., et al. "Evidence for Brain Serotonin-Mediated Control of Carbohydrate Consumption in Normal Weight and Obese Humans," *International Journal of Obesity and Related Metabolic Disorders* 17, no. 9 (Sept. 1993): 513–20.

Poldinger, B.; Calanchini, B; and Schwarz, W. "A Functional-Dimensional

Approach to Depression: Serotonin Deficiency as a Target Syndrome in a Comparison of 5-Hydroxytryptophan and Fluvoxamine," *Psychopathology* 24 (1991): 53–81.

Proietto, J., et al. "Effects of Dexfenfluoramine on Glucose Turnover in Non-Insulin-Dependent Diabetes Mellitus," *Diabetes Research and Clinical Practice* 23, no. 2 (Mar. 1994): 127–34.

Sandyk, Reuven. "L-Tryptophan in Neuropsychiatric Disorders: A Review," *International Journal of Neuroscience* 67 (1992): 127–44.

Spring, Bonnie. "Effects of Foods and Nutrients on the Behavior of Normal Individuals," *Nutrition and the Brain*, vol. 7. New York: Raven Press, 1986.

Wurtman, Judith J., and Suffes, Susan. *The Serotonin Solution: The Potent Substance That Can Help You Stop Bingeing, Lose Weight, and Feel Great.* New York: Ballantine Books, 1996.

Wurtman, R. J., and Wurtman, J. J. "Brain Serotonin, Carbohydrate-Craving, Obesity and Depression," *Obesity Research* 3 Suppl. 4 (Nov. 1995): 477S–80S.

Chapter 11: Your Energy Factor

Alzaid Aus, and Rizza, Robert A. "Insulin Resistance and Its Role in the Pathogenesis of Impaired Glucose Tolerance and Non-Insulin-Dependent Diabetes Mellitus: Perspectives Gained from In Vivo Studies," *Insulin Resistance.* New York: John Wiley & Sons, 1993.

Arner, Peter. "Impact of Exercise on Adipose Tissue Metabolism in Humans," *International Journal of Obesity,* Suppl. 4, no. 19 (1995): 18–21.

Blasi, C. and Jeanrenaud, B. "Insulin Resistance Syndrome: Defective GABA Neuromodulation as a Possible Hereditary Pathogenetic Factor (The 'GABA Hypothesis'), *Medial Hypothesis* 40 (1993): 197–206.

Chan, June M.; Stampfer, Meir J.; Giovannucci, Edward; Gann, Peter H.; Ma, Jing; Wilkinson, Peter; Hennekens, Charles H.; and Pollak, Michael, "Plasma Insulin-Like Growth Factor-I and Prostate Cancer Risk: A Prospective Study," *Science* 279 (Jan. 23, 1998): 563–66.

Duchane, Daniel. *Underground Body Opus Militant Weight Loss and Recomposition.* Carson City, NV: XIPE Press, 1996.

Gianluca, Perseghin; Price, Thomas B.; and Petersen, Kitt F. "Increased Glucose Transport-Phosporylation and Muscle Glycogen Synthesis After Exercise Training in Insulin-Resistant Subjects," *New England Journal of Medicine* 335, no. 18 (Oct. 31, 1996): 1357–62.

Greenspan, Francis S., and Baxter, John D. *Basic and Clinical Endocrinology.* East Norwalk, CT: Appleton & Lange, 1994.

Jeanrenaud, B. "Central Nervous System and Peripheral Abnormalities: Clues to the Understanding of Obesity and NIDDM," *Diabetologia,* Suppl. 2, no. 7 (Sept. 1994): S170–78.

Lauerman, John F. "Diabetes and Yoga Therapy," *Alternative and Complementary Therapies:* (Nov./Dec. 1995): 381–84.

Lee, T. H. "Beneficial Effects of a Mediterranean Diet: A Randomized Trial," *Journal Watch,* 16, no. 23 (Dec. 1, 1996): 184.

Marton, K. I. "Predicting Cardiac Events After Thrombolysis," *Journal Watch* 16, no. 23 (Dec. 1, 1996): 184.

Moses, Alan C., and Abramson, Martin J. "Therapeutic Approaches to Insulin Resistance," *Insulin Resistance.* New York: John Wiley & Sons, 1993.

Ogihara, T., et al. "Enhancement of Insulin Sensitivity by Troglitazone Lowers Blood Pressure in Diabetic Hypertensives," *American Journal of Hypertension* 8, no. 3 (1995): 316–20.

Paolisso, Giuseppe, et al. "Insulin Resistance and Hypertension in the Elderly, Optimal Drug Therapy," *Drugs and Aging* 4, no. 5 (1994): 403–9.

Regelson, William, M.D., and Colman, Carol. *The Super-Hormone Promise: Nature's Antidote to Aging.* New York: Simon and Schuster, 1996.

Sears, Barry. *Mastering the Zone: The Next Step in Achieving Super Health and Permanent Fat Loss.* New York: Regan Books, 1997.

Sears, Barry, and Lawren, Bill, *Enter the Zone: A Dietary Road Map.* New York: Regan Books, 1995.

U.S. Dept. of Health and Human Services, *Healthy People 2000 National Health Promotion and Disease Prevention Objectives.* Boston: Jones and Bartlett, 1992.

Chapter 12: Your Sex Factor

Crenshaw, Theresa L., M.D. *The Alchemy of Love and Lust.* New York: G. P. Putnam's Sons, 1996.

De Lignieres, Bruno. "Transdermal Dihydrotestosterone Treatment of "Andropause," *Annals of Medicine* 25 (1993): 235–41.

Goldin, Barry R., et al. "The Effect of Dietary Fat and Fiber on Serum Estrogen Concentrations in Premenopausal Women Under Controlled Dietary Conditions," *Cancer Supplement* 74, no. 3 (Aug. 1, 1994): 1125–31.

Goodman-Gruen, D., and Barrett-Connor, E. "Total but Not Bioavailable Testosterone Is a Predictor of Central Adiposity in Postmenopausal Women," *International Journal of Obesity and Related Metabolic Disorders* 19, no. 5 (May 1995): 293–98.

Kuiper, Geroge G. J. M.; Carlquist, Mats; and Gustaffsson, Jan-Ake, "Estrogen Is a Male Hormone and Female Hormone," *Science & Medicine* 5, no. 4 (July/Aug. 1998): 36–48.

Kujala, Urho M., M.D.; Kaprio, Jaako, M.D.; Sarna, Seppo, Ph.D.; and Koskenvuo, Markku, M.D., "Relationship of Leisure-Time Physical Activity and Mortality: The Finnish Twin Cohort," *Journal of the American Medical Association* 279 (Feb. 11, 1998): 440–44.

Lieberman, H.; Spring, B.; and Garfield, G. "The Behavioral Effect of Food Constituents: Strategies Used in Studies of Amino Acids, Proteins, Carbohydrates, and Caffeine," *Nutrition Review* 44 (1986): 61–70.

McBride, Gail, and Spencer, Jamie. "Postmenopausal Hormone-Replacement Therapy," *Harvard Health Publications Special Report.* Boston: Harvard Medical School Health Publications Group, 1996.

Ming-Xin, Tang, et al. "Effect of Oestrogent During Menopause on Risk and Age at Onset of Alzheimer's Disease," *Lancet* 348 (Aug. 17, 1996): 429–32.

Morales, A., et al. "Clinical Practice Guidelines for Screening and Monitoring Male Patients Receiving Testosterone Supplementation Therapy," *International Journal of Impotence Research* 8 (1996): 95–97.

Roberts, S. B., "Effects of Aging on Energy Requirements and the Control of Food Intake in Men," *Journals of Gerontology, Series A, Biological Sciences and Medical Sciences* 50 Spec. No. (1995): 101–6.

Rudin, Donald, M.D., and Felix, Clara. *Omega 3 Oils.* New York: Avery Publishing Group, 1996.

Rudy, B. C., and Roberts, R. A., "Gender Differences in Substrate Utilization During Exercise," *Sports Medicine* 17(6) (June 17, 1994): 393–410.

Sahelian, Ray, M.D. *DHEA: A Practical Guide.* New York: Avery Publishing Group, 1996.

———. "Dr. Sahelian's Guide to Natural Hormone Replacement," *Longevity Research Update* 2, no. 1 (1997): 4

Smith, E. P., et al. "Estrogen Resistance Caused by a Mutation in the Estrogen-Receptor Gene in a Man," *New England Journal of Medicine* 331, no. 16 (Oct. 20, 1994): 1056–89.

Swerdloff, R. S., et al. "Effect of Androgens on the Brain and Other Organs During Development and Aging," *Psychoneuroendocrinology* 17, no. 4 (Aug. 1992): 375–83.

Wang, Christine and Swerdloff, Ronald S., "Androgen Replacement Theory," *Annals of Medicine* 29 (1997): 365–70.

Young, Ronald L. "Androgens in Postmenopausal Therapy?" *Menopause Management* (May 1993): 21–24.

Zhang, Yuqing, et al. "Bone Mass and the Risk of Breast Cancer Among Postmenopausal Women," *New England Journal of Medicine* 336, no. 9 (Feb. 27, 1997): 611–17.

Zumoff, Barnett, et al. "Twenty-Four-Hour Mean Plasma Testosterone Concentration Declines with Age in Normal Premenopausal Women," *Journal of Clinical Endocrinology and Metabolism* 80, no. 4 (1995): 1429.

Chapter 13: Your Lifestyle Factor

Berwick, D. M. "Methamphetamine Abuse on the Rise," *Journal Watch* 44 (Dec. 1, 1995): 882–96.

Brett, Allan S., M.D., et al. *Journal Watch* 17, no. 2 (Jan. 15, 1997): 1, 14, 16, 19–20.

Kindermann, W., et al. "Catecholamines, Growth Hormone, Cortisol, Insulin, and Sex Hormones in Anaerobic and Aerobic Exercise," *European Journal of Applied Physiology and Occupational Physiology* 49, no. 3: 389–99.

McEwen, Bruce S. "Re-examination of the Glucocorticoid Hypothesis of Stress and Aging," *Progress in Brain Research*, vol. 93, Elsevier Science Publishers (1992): 365–79.

Michelson, David, M.D., et al. "Bone Mineral Density in Women with Depression," *New England Journal of Medicine* 335, no. 16: 1176–80.

Sapolsky, Robert M. *Why Zebras Don't Get Ulcers: A Guide to Stress, Stress-Related Diseases, and Coping*, New York: W. H. Freeman, 1994.

———. "Why Stress Is Bad for Your Brain," *Science*, 273 (Aug. 9, 1996): 749–50.

Sapolsky, Robert M., et al. "Hippocampal Damage Associated with Prolonged Glucocorticoid Exposure in Primates," *Journal of Neuroscience* 10, no. 4 (Sept. 1990): 2897–2902.

Vita, Anthony J.; Terry, Richard B., Ph.D.; Hubert, Helen B., Ph.D.; and Fries, James, M.D., "Aging, Health Risks, and Cumulative Disability," *The New England Journal of Medicine* 338 (Special Article 1998), 1035–41.

Chapter 14: Your Age Factor

Balin, Arthur K. *Practical Handbook of Human Biologic Age Determination*. Boca Raton, FL: CRC Press, 1994.

Dean, Ward, M.D. *Biological Aging Measurement Clinical Applications*. Los Angeles, CA: The Center for Bio-Gerontology, 1988.

Field, Alison E., et al. "The Relation of Smoking, Age, Relative Weight, and Dietary Intake to Serum Adrenal Steroids, Sex Hormones, and Sex Hormone-Binding Globulin in Middle-Aged Men," *Journal of Clinical Endocrinology and Metabolism* 79, no. 5 (1994): 1310–16.

Goldstein, Irwin, M.D.; Lue, Tom F., M.D.; Padma-Nathan, Harin, M.D.; Rosen, Raymond C., Ph.D.; Steers, William D., M.D.; and Wicker, Pierre A., M.D., for the Sildenafil Study Group, "Oral Sildenafil in the Treatment of Erectile Dysfunction," *The New England Journal of Medicine* 338 (May 14, 1998): 1397–1404.

Grevenstein, J. et al. "Cartilage Changes in Rats Induced by Papain and the Influence of Treatment with N-Acetylglucosamine," *Acta Orthopaedica Belgica* 57 (1991): 157–61.

Harris, Raymond, M.D., and Frankel, Lawrence J. *Guide to Fitness After Fifty*. New York: Plenum Press, 1977.

Padma-Nathan, Harin, et al. "Treatment of Men with Erectile Dysfunction with Transurethral Alprostadil," *New England Journal of Medicine* 336, no. 1 (Jan. 2, 1997): 1–7.

Reichelt, A., et al. "Efficacy and Safety of Intramuscular Glucosamine Sulfate in Osteoarthritis of the Knee, a Randomised, Placebo-Controlled, Double-Blind Study," *Arzneitmittle-Forschung* 44, no. 1 (Jan. 1994): 75–80.

Spirduso, Waneen W. *Physical Dimensions of Aging*. Champaign, IL: Human Kinetics, 1995.

Theodosakis, Jason; Adderly, Brenda; and Fox, Barry. *The Arthritis Cure:*

The Medical Miracle That Can Halt, Reverse, and May Even Cure Osteoarthritis. New York: St. Martin's Press, 1997.

Watson, Ronald R. *Handbook of Nutrition in the Aged.* Boca Raton, FL: CRC Press, 1994.

Zorgniotti, A. W., and Lizza, E. F. "Effect of Large Doses of the Nitric Oxide Precursor, L-Arginine, on Erectile Dysfunction," *International Journal of Impotence Research* 6 (1994): 33–36.

Chapter 16: Antiaging Medicine Chest

Bliznakov, Emile G., M.D., and Hunt, Gerald L. *The Miracle Nutrient: Coenzyme Q_{10},* New York: Bantam Books, 1986.

Carper, Jean. *Stop Aging Now! The Ultimate Plan for Staying Young and Reversing the Aging Process.* New York: HarperPerennial, 1996.

Church and Bowe, *Food Values of Portions Commonly Used,* 16th ed. Philadelphia: J. B. Lippincott Company, 1994.

Dean, Ward, M.D.; Morgenthaler, John; and Fowkes, Steven. *Smart Drugs II The Next Generation: New Drugs and Nutrients to Improve Your Memory and Increase Your Intelligence.* Menlo Park, CA: Health Freedom Publications, 1993.

Klatz, Ronald M., M.D., *Advances in Antiaging Medicine,* vol. 1, New York: Mary Ann Liebert, Inc., 1996.

Lewis, Walter H., and Elvin-Lewis, Memory, P. F. *Medical Botany: Plants Affecting Man's Health.* New York: John Wiley & Sons, 1977.

Morgenthaler, John, and Joy, Dan. *Better Sex Through Chemistry.* Petaluma, CA: Smart Publications, 1994.

Mowrey, Daniel B., *Guaranteed Potency Herbs, Next Generation Herbal Medicine.* New Canaan, CT: Keats Publishing, 1990.

Murray, Michael, and Pizzorno, Joseph. *Encyclopedia of Natural Medicine.* Rocklin, CA: Prima Publishing, 1991.

Ody, Penelope, *The Complete Medicinal Herbal.* New York: Dorling Kindersley, 1993.

Passwater, Richard A. *Lipoic Acid: The Metabolic Antioxidant, the Unique Nutrient That Recharges Energy Levels and the Body's Defenses.* New Canaan, CT: Keats Publishing, 1995.

———. *The New Superantioxidant-Plus: The Amazing Story of Pycnogenol, Free-Radical Antagonist and Vitamin C Potentiator.* New Canaan, CT: Keats Publishing, 1992.

Sahelian, Ray, M.D. *Pregnenolone: A Practical Guide.* Marina del Rey, CA: Melatonin/DHEA Research Institute, 1996.

Sahelian, Ray, M.D., and Tuttle, David. *Creatine, Nature's Muscle Builder.* New York: Avery Publishing Group, 1997.

Shabert, Judy, M.D., and Erlich, Nancy. *The Ultimate Nutrient Glutamine.* New York: Avery Publishing Group, 1994.

Watt, Bernice K., et al. *Handbook of the Nutritional Contents of Foods.* New York: Dover Publications, 1975.

Werbach, Melvin R., M.D. *Nutritional Influences on Illness: A Sourcebook of*

Clinical Research. Tarzana, CA: Third Line Press, 1988.

Werbach, Melvin R., M.D. and Murray, Michael T., M.D. *Botanical Influences on Illness: A Sourcebook of Clinical Research*. Tarzana, CA: Third Line Press, 1994.

Bland, Jeffrey, Ph.D. "Dietary Fibers: Insoluble and Soluble," *Technical Bulletins*. Educational/Technical Focus. GIG Harbor, WA: HealthComm International, Inc. 1995.

Chapter 17: Food Choices

Murray, Michael. *The Healing Power of Herbs*. Rocklin, CA: Prima Publishing, 1995.

————. *Encyclopedia of Nutritional Supplements: The Essential Guide for Improving Your Health Naturally*. Rocklin, CA: Prima Publishing, 1996.

Epilogue: Antiaging Medicine in the Twenty-first Century

Dilbert, M. S., et al. "Suicide Gene Therapy for Plasma Cell Tumors," *Blood* 88, no. 6 (Sept. 15, 1996): 2192–2200.

Patel, P. I. "Identification of Disease Genes and Somatic Gene Therapy: An Overview and Prospects for the Aged," *Journal of Gerontology* 48, no. 3 (May 1993): B80–85.

Singh, N., and Anand, S. "Apoptosis in Health and Disease," *Indian Journal of Physiology and Pharmacology* 39, no. 2 (Apr. 1995): 1–4.

Sinkovics, J., and Horvath, J. "Apoptosis by Genetic Engineering," *Leukemia* 1, no. 8 (Apr. 1994): S98–102.

Zhang, L., et al. "Depth-Targeted Efficient Gene Delivery and Expression in the Skin by Pulsing Electric Fields: An Approach to Gene Therapy of Skin Aging and Other Diseases," *Biochemical and Biophysical Research Communications* 220, no. 3 (Mar. 27, 1996): 633–36.

Index